THE F*CK
THOUGHTS
THAT
F*CK
YOU UP

... and how to fix them

REWIRE HOW YOU THINK IN SIX WEEKS WITH REBT

DANIEL FRYER

Vermilion
LONDON

1 3 5 7 9 10 8 6 4 2

Published in 2019 by Vermilion an imprint of Ebury Publishing,
20 Vauxhall Bridge Road,
London SW1V 2SA

Vermilion is part of the Penguin Random House group of companies
whose addresses can be found at global.penguinrandomhouse.com

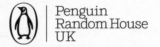

Penguin
Random House
UK

First published by Vermilion in 2019

www.penguin.co.uk

A CIP catalogue record for this book is available from the British Library

ISBN 9781785042843

Typeset in 11.5/16.1 pt Slate Std
by Integra Software Services Pvt. Ltd, Pondicherry

Printed and bound in Great Britain by Clays Ltd, Elcograf S.p.A.

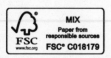

For my Mum
infamy, of sorts

Contents

No one and nothing is completely useless, rubbish, worthless or a failure. Here you will not only learn to never use the term self-esteem again, you'll also learn why it's better to never use that term again. Seriously, just drop it

Part Two: The Four Thoughts That Will Fix Them

This is a much more rational expression of a desire for something. It's perfectly reasonable to wish, hope or want for something, as long as you accept that you live in a world where you don't always get it. Sad, but true

Would you like to see problems in their true perspective, without ever blowing them out of proportion or making them worse than they actually are? You would? Jolly good, as this is the chapter where you get to do that

Or, how to recover quickly from life's many difficulties and debacles. Here you will develop mental and emotional toughness in the face of adversity and discover that you have coped with way more than you ever gave yourself credit for

Unconditional Acceptance   120

You are a worthwhile, fallible human being. You are
sufficient as is. Yes, you are. So is everybody else. Things
are worthwhile and fallible too. Find out why believing
this is both good for self-confidence and great for giving
up the grudge-holding

Part Three: Rewire How You Think in Just Six Weeks With Rational Emotive Behaviour Therapy

WEEK ONE: REBT: A Cunning Plan   137

Getting to grips with both Rational Emotive Behaviour
Therapy and the ABCDE model of psychological
health, because this particular therapy has both a
philosophy and a structure. Not a lot of therapies
can say that

WEEK TWO: How to Pick and Pick Apart a Problem   158

Nothing is as complicated as it seems, at least not
according to the ABCDE model of psychological
health – we're not just identifying the thoughts
that fuck you up, but the dysfunctional emotions
and behaviours they can trigger too

WEEK THREE: Questioning the Validity of Your Thoughts   194

Promoting intellectual understanding and learning
to question the validity of your thoughts. Not as
dangerous as it sounds

An Introduction

The happiness of your life depends upon the quality of your thoughts.

Marcus Aurelius

People that meet me think me very calm and placid, unflappable even. People that know me remember the short-tempered and impatient little grumpus[1] that I was before I ever studied and practised psychotherapy, especially one form of psychotherapy in particular.

Very, very few people that remember me as that grumpus know that I once raced in my car after a motorist I had just given way to, cut them up, forced them to a standstill in the middle of the road, and then ran up to their car and, hammering heavily on the driver's side window, screamed at them very loudly, 'The next time someone lets you pass, you say thank you!'

---

[1] A grumpus, according to the Urban Dictionary, is a terminally grumpy person, often genetic; it can be modified for various states of grumpity.

1

The driver nodded vigorously in terrified acquiescence and so I walked back to my car, got in and drove away calmly, albeit with a thumping headache from my angry outburst.

It was not my finest moment.

In my defence, they were the third such motorist that I had given way to on the same long, narrow stretch of road, and I was feeling more than a little aggrieved. But, that was a long time ago and, thankfully, that excellent form of therapy has stood me in good stead, guiding me through many frustrating situations over the years.

I first came to Rational Emotive Behaviour Therapy (REBT) in 2005. Perhaps unsurprisingly, I learnt about it on a course I was studying (me being a practising therapist and all).

Before that, I worked in journalism and publishing, so I really do know a thing or two about stress, pressure and deadlines. Far more than was probably healthy at the time. I thought therapy would be more fulfilling for me. Surprisingly, it was. I also used to work in London (stressful) and then moved to Bristol a few years ago (not-so-stressful). Somewhere along the line I acquired a dog. She's a Staffy; a rescue from Battersea Dogs and Cats Home, and I accidentally turned her into a working therapy dog. And a famous one at that. She has appeared in articles and features of her own. She plays it down but, secretly, I think she enjoys all the attention.

But back then, I'd been working as a hypnotherapist for a little over a year and I wanted to build on and consolidate my learning. REBT is a very structured and goal-orientated form of psychotherapy that looks at challenging your disturbing thoughts about any given situation and replacing them with more helpful alternatives. Solution-focused and practical, it looks at where you are and where you want to be and then gives you the tools to help get you there.

The tutors on the course were practising therapists themselves. Each week they would explain a different aspect of the therapy and explore a different topic. They would often ask for volunteers from the class to come up to the front and aid them in demonstrating various aspects and practices of the therapy.

'Pick a real problem to work through,' the tutors would say. 'Not only will you be able to focus on your own personal development, but you'll be able to experience first-hand just how effective this particular form of therapy is.'

But the volunteers never offered up any real problems. They were too nervous. They made their problems up, or they offered pseudo-problems; they even role-played other people's problems. You could tell.

One day, a student offered himself up for demonstration purposes; there he sat at the front of the class as the tutor asked him what he would like to work on.

'Well,' he said slowly, staring off into the middle distance and clearly reflecting deeply on exactly what it was that he wanted to volunteer. 'I don't always clean my fish tank out on time and I'd like to know why.'

The audience groaned and the tutor exclaimed, 'Oh for god's sake! No one is ever going to pay you good money to work on that as a problem. Has anyone got any actual problems they want to work on?'

Tentatively, my hand went up.

'What have you got for me?' said tutor enquired.

'An anger-management issue,' said I.

The tutor's face lit up with glee. 'What is it?' he asked, as twenty pairs of student eyeballs zeroed in on me.

'I don't like crowded places,' I said. 'I don't like traffic jams or rush hours. I don't like people that cut me up, either on foot or in cars. I don't like crowded train platforms or crowded trains, I don't like shopping malls or concert halls, and I don't like football matches or festivals. I don't even like people who walk too slowly. Basically, I don't like anywhere and every-where a large amount of people gather, either to go in, or congregate in, or leave.'

'And what makes you think this is an unhealthy anger-management problem rather than just, say, normal frustration?' he asked.

'Well,' I said, my face reddening a little, 'I mutter under my breath a lot. I can shout and swear at people a whole lot, and I will often growl at people like a bear. If I'm really angry, I will physically grab them and shove them out of my way and, if I'm really, really angry, I will do all of the above.'

'Hot damn,' he said. 'That's anger. Please come up to the front.'

He asked me a few more questions about my crowded places anger-management issue and, in a very short space of time, managed to deduce exactly what it was that I was getting angry about. From there, using the tools and tech-niques of REBT, he worked out the four thoughts that were fucking me up very quickly indeed.

I worked on those thoughts continuously over the duration of the course and, to the relief of crowds of people everywhere,

I never, ever muttered, shouted, swore, growled, grabbed or hammered on car windows again.[2]

But, what exactly is Rational Emotive Behaviour Therapy, what does it achieve, and how can it help you think, feel and act in a more appropriate way?

In a slight case of acronym overkill, REBT is a form of Cognitive Behaviour Therapy (CBT) that takes a simple-yet-cunning approach to mental wellness, where Activating events (A) trigger Beliefs (B) that cause Consequences (C). You Dispute (D) your beliefs vigorously and repeatedly, which leads to an Effective rational outlook (E) to that original activating event. This is known as the ABCDE model of psychological health, and I'll be explaining it in greater detail later on.

This model allows you to identify and challenge unhealthy thoughts that are triggering unhelpful emotions and behaviours while, at the same time, helping you to formulate and reinforce a series of more healthy thoughts that will trigger more helpful emotions and behaviours.

As beliefs at 'B', there are four types of unhealthy cognition (the thoughts that can fuck you up) and four healthy, rational equivalents than can help keep you calm in the face of adversity – which we'll explore in Parts One and Two of the book.[3]

Pioneered and developed in the mid-1950s by a New York psychotherapist called Albert Ellis, REBT predates the more commonly practised form of CBT (developed by the

---

[2] Well, not exactly never, more sort of never; well, almost never; never(ish). An occasional blip really is just par for the course. Honest. As you will soon discover.

[3] Or unfuck you.

psychiatrist Aaron T. Beck) by about 10 years. Albert Ellis is sadly deceased (he passed away in 2007), but his therapy remains. He was, and is still considered, an unsung hero in the therapy world. In a 1982 professional survey of American and Canadian psychologists, he was rated as the second most influential psychotherapist in history. Freud came in at number three.

Back in the humble beginnings of both, REBT was known as Rational Therapy (RT) and CBT was known as Cognitive Therapy (CT). Later, they both became two separate but similar branches of the same CBT tree. CBT therapists rarely clarify whether you are getting the Beck model or the Ellis model when they are delivering your therapy but, generally speaking, it's the Beck model you are getting. Which is a shame really, because REBT has a philosophy and a structure that is easy to explain, elegant to execute and bloody brilliant at bringing you back from the brink of anger, anxiety, depression and a whole host of other unhealthy negative emotions and behaviours.

This book firmly waves the flag for this form of CBT. It's a therapy that few people outside the realms of psychotherapy have heard of (including several people who have actually had it as their main form of therapy). It is widely considered to be the first form of CBT and, for me personally, it is the much more effective form of CBT. Other people and other therapists are free to disagree.

As with all of the cognitive behavioural therapies, REBT is an evidence-based practice. This means that, over the years, many studies and experiments have successfully demonstrated how effective it is in treating a wide range of conditions.

Eight unhealthy negative emotional problems are discussed in this book, but it's also excellent at treating behavioural issues as well, such as addictions and all those bad habits that you just can't seem to break. In fact, simply typing the term 'REBT' into Google Scholar will yield a dazzling array of results for you to get your academic teeth into.[4]

Over the years, seeing people individually and in group therapy settings, I've always been impressed with the changes people have made for the better; how they have dealt with vexing situations and challenging problems more effectively by using REBT. More than a fair few people have said to me things along the lines of, 'I wish I had come to this style of therapy sooner,' or, 'I wish I'd know about this therapy years ago.'

There are many books on REBT and yet, not many people are aware of this style of therapy. Hence this book, which doesn't just sing this form of CBT's praises, it shouts them out loud. It screams, 'Look at REBT! It's magnificent! If you want to stop doing your head in; if you want to stop doing other people's heads in, it can really help you!' And then, it shows you how to do that. And it does so in three parts.

Part One introduces you to the four thoughts that fuck you up. They are four specific types of unhealthy belief that, according to REBT, lie at the heart of nearly all types of psychological disturbance.

Part Two will discuss the four rational alternatives that stop you from fucking yourself up, and do so by promoting psychological wellbeing.

---

[4] If you have academic teeth, that is. Or dentures.

7

Together, these two sections invite you to look at life, and all of its problems and challenges, in a whole new way; they show you how to make a general, philosophical shift in the way you look at things.

The examples used in the first two parts of this book are both similar and linked, which may seem a little repetitive, but it is done with good reason. Firstly, repetition is key (more of that later); and, secondly, in order to highlight how you can systematically weaken an unhealthy set of beliefs and strengthen the healthier alternatives, I comprehensively attack a similar series of beliefs throughout.

Part Three is where we get down to the nitty-gritty: this book will help you work through a specific emotional problem in just six weeks.

Yes, you read that right. In just six sessions (if you apply yourself diligently) you could rewire your brain so that you react in a totally different way to a problem or challenge.

But, there are two conditions attached. Firstly, the problem needs to be as specific as possible and, secondly, it should be mildly to moderately disturbing (as opposed to severely disturbing in which case I would recommend working directly with a therapist). For example, social anxiety is a specific problem, as is performance anxiety, as is depression over losing a job or a relationship. Getting angry with a certain person or in a certain situation also counts, as does being jealous of your partner or insecure in your relationship.

Six sessions is a magic number favoured by nearly all health insurance companies, mainly because 'six sessions' is buried somewhere among National Institute of Clinical Excellence (NICE) guidelines. NICE is part of the National Health Service

(NHS) and is the organisation that provides guidance and advice that helps improve health and social care. It recognises six sessions as appropriate in treating a wide range of specific conditions at the mild to moderate end of the spectrum.[5] Also, from personal experience, I have helped many, many people gain control of specific anxiety, anger-management, depression and jealousy problems in just six sessions.

There's a caveat attached to those two conditions. If you have a clinical condition (such as clinical depression), or if you are dealing with a current or recent trauma, it would be best to seek the services of a professional, rather than rely on this book.

Clinical conditions are not the result of your beliefs, but are down to a complicated set of factors that include environment, circumstance, brain chemistry and more. It's not that this book can't help you; it's just that the approach would be slightly different. Also, this book uses humour to get its message across. It's not used to belittle or demean what you are going through, but to help you move on from it. Humour is an excellent therapeutic tool, however, it's not the best approach to use with someone who is in the midst of a severe episode of, say, clinical depression.

Similarly, REBT can be used to resolve and move on from trauma. However, it's for people who are 'stuck', for those who find it difficult to move on from something that

---

[5] REBT and CBT are known as 'brief' therapies; this means sessions last from weeks to months, as opposed to years. Six months of REBT or CBT would be considered brief; so six sessions is very brief indeed.

happened some time ago. If the traumatic incident is a recent event, then counselling with a trained professional would be much better for you than this book. A counsellor will provide you with a safe space in which to explore and process your emotions. Again, humour can help, but a little later on in the process. In the immediacy of something traumatic, or shocking, humour can seem seriously at odds with the very real and valid emotions you are experiencing. This also applies to grief. Following bereavement, grief counselling would be a better fit for you than this book.

So, clinical conditions and recent trauma aside, if you think you can identify a specific problem, at the preferably mild to moderate end of the spectrum, then please read on. If not, please seek out the services of a professional.

Part Three of this book takes a step-by-step approach and will help you to identify and work upon your specific problem until you have effected a solution that works for you.

Weeks One to Six in this approach will require 'homework'. There will be things to read, write, think about and do. I've left space for you to write things down in those chapters, but some people don't like defacing their books in such a way. Some even consider it sacrilegious to do so. If you are one of them, you might want to buy a notebook or journal before you get to this part of the book. There are also forms that you can download from my website: www.danielfryer.com.

This book is stuffed full of anecdotes (some of them deliberately repetitive and/or connected), not only from my time working on my own personal anger-management issue, but from nearly fifteen years of practising REBT on both myself and others. And, fear not, for the names have been changed to protect the innocent. Also, I don't use any names.[6]

With this book, you will learn how to adapt flexibly to challenging situations, see things in their true perspective (without blowing them out of proportion or magnifying the difficulty) and learn to accept yourself and other people as pretty awesome, but slightly flawed, individuals.

In doing so, I can't promise less stress in your life, but I can promise that you will deal with the stress you do have in a much more effective fashion. In short, you'll learn how to stop fucking yourself up in the face of adversity. And when it comes to the four thoughts that fuck you up, nothing will fuck you up quite like a demand for something . . .

Want to meet one?

---

[6] Except for once or twice.

PART ONE

THE FOUR THOUGHTS THAT F*CK YOU UP

Dogmatic Demands

The mature person meets the demands of life, while the immature person demands that life meet their demands.

Henry Cloud

When it comes to the four thoughts that fuck you up, Public Enemy Number One is the 'Dogmatic Demand'. Behind any emotional or behavioural problem that disturbs you (i.e., if you are thinking and feeling and acting in ways that you don't like, but don't seem to be able to change), there is a demand for something. But, what exactly is a demand?

In REBT a 'demand' has one specific meaning: it is a rigid, dogmatic belief that disturbs you. Demands take the form of words such as 'must' and 'mustn't', 'should' and 'shouldn't', and 'got to' and 'have to'. And by rigid and dogmatic, I mean you are holding a belief that you think is undeniably and absolutely true. It's an inflexible, inviolable law that you hold in your head, one that cannot ever be broken (or else, calamity!). You are demanding one thing and one thing only. It's a belief so absolute that no other option is ever allowed. Sounds pretty extreme, right?

It's usually the rigid expression of a desire for something. So, 'I would like to have' becomes 'I must have' and that can be applied to anything and affect everything. If you have an unreasonable response to a person, a situation or whatever, then behind that unreasonable response there is a demand for something. Later on, in Part Three of this book, I'll be giving a framework to hang this notion off but, for now, all you need to know is, that when it comes to the four thoughts that fuck you up, the demand is the primary thing.

For instance, let's say that I have a thing about time keeping – a desire for punctuality. And, let's say that, behind that desire, I have formulated the rigid, absolutist belief that I must be on time for everything. And I mean it absolutely, as in all the time, every time, no matter what, end of discussion.

This makes it a dogmatic demand, in that it is the rigid expression of the desire to be on time for everything. It's perfectly fine to *want* to be on time, that's not the problem. The problem is my belief: 'I *must* be on time for everything'.

A rigid demand messes you up on several levels. First of all it's often unrealistic. It's so rigid and absolute that there's no wiggle room in there; there is literally only the one option. Which is crazy, because it doesn't take into account any delay. Because, sometimes (or often, actually), there are delays. Right now, for example, as I am typing this particular chapter, I am on a Bristol Temple Meads to London Paddington train that is delayed.[1]

---

[1] Depending on your point of view, this is either irony or synchronicity in action.

Demands are also illogical. It's perfectly fine to be the sort of person who likes to be on time, but it is not logical to insist that you must be, just because you want to be.

Finally, demands do not help you; instead they disturb you, they fuck you up. They mess with your head. Demanding that you must be on time for everything does not change the fact that you will inevitably be delayed from time to time, but it does mean that you won't cope with the delays very well at all.

This makes them irrational and, by that we mean unhelpful, in that they don't give you good psychological results (i.e., they make you angry, or anxious, or depressed, and so on), and they don't help you achieve your goals. In short, they fuck you up because they are rigid and dogmatic: they don't fit in with the reality of the situation, they don't make logical sense and they don't help you.

Before I delve a little deeper into the dysfunctional world of demands, I want to talk about all the demands that don't mess you up because, outside the world of REBT and the realm of your head, words like 'must' and 'should' are thrown around with regular and non-freaky abandon.

Demands That Don't Disturb You

First up, we have empirical demands such as the inviolable laws of science that cannot be broken. My favourite one is the law of gravity, because it contains an actual demand, namely that 'what goes up must come down'. That law is not going to disturb you, or anyone else for that matter; it's just a statement of fact. Here, on planet Earth, without the aid of physics and about a million pounds of rocket fuel, what goes up always comes back down.

Now, let's say I know you socially, and that you and I are enjoying a walk in the sunshine and are having a nice chat. We pass an al fresco coffee stand and I suddenly exclaim, 'Oh my god, you simply must have the salted caramel macchiato.'

Firstly, you might accuse me of being a member of the pampered, liberal bourgeoisie for even knowing of such a thing, let alone what it actually tastes like but secondly, and more importantly, there's that word 'must' again. But, I'm certainly not going to disturb anyone with my demand, I'm simply making a recommendation: try that particular type of coffee, it's a bit lovely, is what I'm saying.

Still sticking with a 'knowing you socially' scenario, let's imagine you invite me round for dinner, only I'm slightly late. You know I set out by car ages ago and yet you haven't heard from me, so you give me a call. 'Sorry,' I say. 'Traffic held me up. But, it's okay now. I should be there in about 20 minutes or so if things remain clear.' Again, I've made a demand (in this instance, 'should') but, again, not one that disturbs either party. Instead, I'm making a prediction. As long as the roads remain congestion-free, I think I will be there soon.

We also have what are known as 'ideal demands'. In an ideal world, people wouldn't litter; in an ideal world people wouldn't kill other people, there wouldn't be any homelessness and all things would be fair and equal for all of us. But, sadly we don't live in an ideal world. People litter, people kill, homelessness is an ever-growing problem and the world is neither fair, nor equal. However, people do express their ideals in conversation and that is perfectly fine and dandy.

There is no need to leap on them and say, 'Ah-ha, that's a rigid belief and you must not express it.'[2]

However, the most common demand issued on a daily basis is known as a conditional demand: ABC must happen in order for XYZ to take place. Let's say I commute to work by train, as many of us do. And let's say that I have that belief of 'I must be on time for everything'. As you know, trains are not the most reliable of things; at least not in the UK. Now imagine I travel with a notoriously bad operator, not known for its punctuality record. With this belief, I am going to be anxious before I even get on the train. In fact, I'm probably going to become the sort of person that gets on a train way earlier than the one I need, just to be on the safe side. I'm also likely to be very disturbed each and every time that train seems to slow down or stop.

But, if I tell you that I must be on time in order to get to an important meeting, or to a job interview that starts at 2pm prompt why, then, it's conditional: ABC (being on time) must happen in order for XYZ (getting to that important meeting or to that job interview on time) to occur. It's a statement of fact.

Life and other people place lots of conditional demands on you that impact upon your time, your social life, your ability to plan and even your wellbeing, but it's up to you whether you disturb yourself about those conditions or not.

So, the demands that don't disturb you include empirical demands, recommendations, predictions, ideal demands and conditional demands. You can make those and accept those from others as much or as little as you wish.

---

[2] You telling someone they must not express something, however, is a rigid demand. Naughty you.

Back To The Demands That Do Disturb You

Must and mustn't; should and shouldn't; got to and have to. Collectively these are known as demands, they are beliefs that disturb you, that cause problems such as anxiety and depression, because they are rigid, unrealistic, illogical and unhelpful.

In terms of REBT and the four thoughts that mess you up, these really are the first type that you need to look out for. Behind your angry outburst, there is a demand for something; behind your panic attack, there is a demand for something. Behind your depressive episodes, your jealous rages, your addictions and more, there are demands for things.

'Cherchez le must,' said Albert Ellis, who wasn't even French: always look for the demand. If you are thinking, feeling and acting in ways that you don't like, but don't seem to be able to change: always look for the demand. In fact, from now on, whenever you are thinking, feeling or acting irrationally, try to take a step back and think, 'What is it that I am demanding?'

For example, if you argue with your partner about doing the dishes and are angry at their lack of respect, you will have the demand 'my partner must respect me'. If you get anxious when talking to your boss and are worried about looking like a fool in front of them, you will have the demand 'I must not look like a fool in front of my boss'. If you have a lift phobia and your biggest fear is 'getting stuck in a lift', then your demand would be 'I must not get stuck in a lift'.

If you are an all-or-nothing perfectionist, then you have a demand for everything to be perfect; if you freak out whenever things aren't completely under your control, you have a demand to be in control, if you get anxious at the mere thought of getting anxious, then you have the demand not to get anxious. I could go on, but I hope I'm getting the point across.

To work out what you are demanding, try and identify what is really disturbing you in any given situation. For instance, if you are angry with a partner, or a colleague, ask yourself, 'What is it I am really, really angry about here?' If you are depressed about something, ask yourself, 'What is it that depresses me the most about this situation?' Once you have identified the thing that disturbs you the most, stick a demand word in there and, voilà, you have your unhealthy belief. And, once you have your unhealthy belief, you can challenge it.

Back when I first volunteered in the classroom all those years ago, when I first brought up my 'love' of crowds and crowded spaces in a therapeutic setting, the thing that angered me the most (as the tutor quickly ascertained) was 'other people getting in my way'. I really, really didn't like that when it happened. The thing that made me angry though was my belief; my desire made absolute, the rigid expression of that want. In short, the thought that fucked me up was the demand that 'other people must not get in my way'.[3]

And I really meant it: everywhere, all the time.

---

[3] This wasn't the only problem in life I've needed to work on using REBT, or even the most disturbing. It was, however, the only problem I was willing to voice in front of twenty-or-so very curious fellow students.

Challenging Your Demands

In REBT we learn to challenge our beliefs, both the unhealthy and the healthy. We challenge our unhealthy beliefs to weaken them to the point of collapse, and strengthen the healthy beliefs so we have something bright and shiny and good for us to replace the unhealthy ones with when they do collapse. Nature abhors a vacuum after all and if you don't replace something unhealthy with something healthy, something equally unhealthy, or worse even, could creep in.

In REBT, challenging your beliefs is known as 'disputing'. Earlier, I said that demands were unrealistic, that they didn't make sense and that they didn't help you. Disputing is REBT putting its money where its mouth is.

There are many methods for challenging your beliefs but disputing primarily takes the form of challenging your beliefs with three questions. Those questions are:

1. 'Is this belief true?'
2. 'Does this belief make sense?'
3. 'Does this belief help me?'

Truth and sense and helpfulness: or – if you want to be fancy about it – empirical, logical and pragmatic questions.

Empirical means to be based on (or concerned with, or verifiable by) observation or experience, while logical means according to the rules of logic or formal argument, or something characterised by or capable of clear, sound reasoning. Finally, pragmatic means dealing with things sensibly and realistically.

So, the 'is it true?' question is a science question; it wants proof, it wants evidence. Whatever answer you give, whether it is 'yes, that belief is true' or 'no, that belief is false', you are going to have to back up your answer with evidence.

The 'does it make sense?' question is asking for sound reasoning, or for a hefty dose of common sense. Just because I think <insert thing here> does it logically follow that <insert conclusion here>?

Finally, the 'does it help me?' question is, hopefully, the most obvious member of the trio. If you're reading this book, you most probably have a reason for doing so, a therapeutic or psychological goal in mind. So, you simply ask yourself, 'Does this belief help me behave sensibly or realistically? Does my belief help me achieve that goal?'

These questions might sound simple and, on one level they are. But, they are also very rational, very objective questions – questions that cut right through to the heart of the matter. And, because they are so rational, they are used everywhere; not just in therapy. Maths, science, philosophy, law and debating teams up and down the country, anywhere anyone has a point of view or a statement to uphold, can be challenged with these questions.

Let's say I am a scientist, and I have just successfully run an experiment that revolutionises our understanding of Einstein's theory of relativity. I'm going to think myself pretty clever, aren't I? More importantly, I'm going to want to get my experiment down on paper and published in a journal. So I take my results to my peers. The first thing they are going to ask for is the evidence. It I don't have any, or my evidence is flawed, I'm stuffed. But, if I can provide good, solid evidence, then I'm over the first hurdle. So the next attack is logical. Does my research make sense? Does my conclusion logically follow from my premise? If the answer is no, I will not be published. But, if my ideas flow logically, one to the other, from the beginning to the end, then I've cleared another hurdle. Finally, we have the pragmatic question. Does my experiment help; does it expand on what's gone before; does it add anything new? If it doesn't, I'm going home with my tail between my legs but, if it does add something new, if it goes beyond what Einstein originally proposed, then we are good to go. So, let's apply that way of thinking to a demand.

Demands Are Not True: Because You Will Have Evidence To The Contrary

Let's look at the demand 'I must be on time for everything'. How can that be true? Delays occur every single day, delays on trains, delays on buses and delays on coaches; delays due to breakdowns or congested traffic at a standstill, even delays because your nearest and dearest couldn't quite get themselves into gear that day. If you've ever been held up or delayed for any reason, if you have ever been late for an appointment, then the demand 'I must be on time for everything' is not true. Your delay, the fact that you have been late, is the evidence.

When asked by me if 'I must be on time for everything' is true, people often say 'yes'. And, as evidence to back up their answer, they cite examples such as: 'there could be negative consequences to my delay', 'my boss doesn't like it when I'm late', 'I don't like it when I'm late' or 'I get really frustrated when I am delayed'. These things don't prove the 'must' to be true though. However, they do highlight why you, personally, prefer to be on time.

Some have also tried to prove 'I must be on time for everything' as true by claiming that their boss demands that they have to be in on time. But, this means that either your boss is holding an unhealthy dogmatic demand or they are issuing you with a factual conditional demand. If it's the latter, they are saying you must be on time or else. (Or else I will get angry, or else there will be lost time, or else I will deduct your wages, or else I am making you work late, and so on.)

You are not responsible for how your boss thinks, or feels or acts. You are not responsible for the beliefs they hold (rational or otherwise). You are only responsible for how you think, feel and act in the face of your boss's behaviour.

Their dogmatic demand of you (if that is what they are making) is not true. Your demand of you is not true: no rigid, dogmatic demand anyone could ever make can ever be true. Just take the following example . . .

I'm bald. (Bear with me on this.) I started losing my hair in my late teens. By my mid-twenties I gave up the ghost and cropped my hair really short. Perhaps it's because I have a picture of myself on my website, perhaps not, but over the years I have had many, many young bald or balding men come to see me for therapy, anxious and depressed and lacking in confidence because of their lack of hair.

'But I shouldn't be bald!' many of them have cried out in my therapy room. 'My dad wasn't bald, my granddad wasn't bald; so I shouldn't be bald!' Sadly, their big, bald heads – heads that often contained even less hair than mine – in men younger than I – were themselves the evidence that that particular demand was simply not true.

Empirical demands are true. Take my favourite, the law of gravity, or 'what goes up must come down'. If I throw a ball up in the air, it will come down. If I throw it up in the air a hundred times or a gazillion times, it will come down every single time. I could tell you I threw it up in the air last week and I could tell you I am going to throw it up in the air next week. It always came down; it always will come down, 100 per cent of the time. Here, on planet Earth, it is an inviolable law.

If you are demanding respect then you must be able to evidence 100 per cent respect, 100 per cent of the time. If you can't do that, the demand is not true. If you are demanding to be in control, then you must be able to evidence 100 per cent control 100 per cent of the time, and that means you cannot give one single example of ever having had control slip from your grasp. Can't do it, can you?

You can demand that lifts must not get stuck as much as you like, but that doesn't prevent them from getting stuck. And, chances are, if you've ever been on board one then you too have been stuck in a lift at some point in your life. There isn't a single demand that can't be disproved by providing evidence to the contrary.

The laws of the land and biblical laws are not absolute. They are conditional. A big law (both land wise and biblically) is that you mustn't kill people. As a demand, it can't be true because, sadly and regrettably, people get murdered (or are killed accidentally) every single day. What the law of the land is actually saying is that you must not kill people, or else you will be thrown into prison.[4]

Demands Don't Make Sense: That's Not The Way The World Works

Do you know the story of Aladdin and the lamp? It's a Middle Eastern folktale and one of the stories from The *Book of One Thousand and One Nights (The Arabian Nights)*. Very briefly, among his many adventures, loveable street urchin Aladdin finds a magic lamp. When he rubs the lamp, a genie appears and grants him three boons.

'Your wish is my command,' the genie says.

Just think what you could wish for if you had such a lamp.

'I want to win the lottery,' you say. And, with a click of its fingers, the genie makes it happen. Look at you, luxuriating in all that cash.

'I want a brand new Aston Martin DB9,' you say. And click! The genie makes it happen. And there you are, putting pedal to the sleek and sexy metal on the highway.

'I want to be on time,' you say, 'for everything,' you add, and click! The genie makes it happen. And there you are, safe and sure in the knowledge that you will never, ever be delayed again.

Can you imagine never wanting for anything ever again? Depending on your point of view, that would either be complete heaven, or total hell. But the point here is this: there is no genie, there is no lamp and your wish is no one's command.

---

[4] If you are caught, that is.

You do not get what you want just by wishing it: the world just doesn't work like that.

It makes no logical sense to say you must have a thing, just because you would like to have a thing. You might wish to win the lottery, but that doesn't necessarily mean that you must win it. And you probably won't, as it is a game of chance after all: the wish is one thing, but the demand is another. Logically the two don't connect. There are just too many factors between them. You've got to buy a ticket, for starters.

You might wish for a brand new Aston Martin DB9, but just because you wish for it, it doesn't logically follow that you must have it. They are two different things and logically they don't connect. Again there are just too many factors between the two: can you afford the deposit, the monthly repayments, the insurance and the running costs?[5]

It's the same with any demand. Don't forget that a demand is just the rigid expression of a *desire* for something. It's okay to want to be on time, to like to be in control, to wish for more respect from your partner or for more hair on your head than you currently display but, just because you wish for these things, it does not logically follow that you must have them.

When you hold a dogmatic demand, you are not demonstrating sound, logical reasoning at all.

Demands Don't Help You: Just Look At What You Get

All a rigid demand does is make you react in ways that aren't helpful to yourself and others. If you demand to be on time

---

[5] Guess what I'm buying if this book is a bestselling success?

for everything, all you will do when faced with an inevitable delay is freak out about it. You might, in all probability, be one of those people who doesn't just arrive early, but who arrives irrationally early for things. Like, two hours early, just to be safe. You might be like one of the people I'm watching on the train right now as I write this, swearing under your breath, or berating the on-board services manager, or venting your frustrations on social media or ranting down your phone thusly: 'Yes, Tom – it's bloody well happened again. I know it'll be fucking chaos without me, you'll just have to soldier on.'[6]

If you have a test coming up, and you're demanding that you must pass your test, you will make yourself anxious; you will revise poorly, sleep badly and perform less well come the day. (If you perform at all, as we've all seen people flee their exams in tears.)

You might demand more respect from your partner, but when you don't get it all you do is get all angry and shouty. You then get involved in an argument which ends up with nobody respecting anybody. You might demand perfection but, instead of being motivated to do well, you are driven by a fear of failure; you're operating on adrenaline and, if you fail to hit your mark, you could plunge into despair. It's all or nothing for you. And, if you're demanding to be in control of everything, all the time, then all that does is turn you into a crazy, control freak person, secretly afraid that you've turned out just like your mother.[7]

---

[6] This actually happened on my train journey.

[7] You know who you are.

My anger-provoking demand of 'other people must not get in my way' was not true. Every single example of every single person that bumped into me, or trod on my feet, or stood stock still right in front of me for no apparent reason, or stopped to have a chat in the doorway of a really busy shop just as I was walking through it, or who knocked my drink all over me or barged right past me was proof that the demand just wasn't true.

And while it made perfect sense for me to prefer other people to not get in my way, it made no sense to conclude that they mustn't. (I really do prefer it though. If I had my way, no one would travel when I travelled and all shops would mysteriously empty whenever I entered them.) While this is a nice idea, it does not make for sound reasoning. The wish is one thing but the demand is another.

Finally, that belief did not help me. It made me angry, it made me shout and swear and growl and grab people which, I'm told, is not appropriate behaviour, even though it felt totally justifiable at the time.

And there you have it. Dogmatic demands are rigid beliefs that disturb you (in that they cause emotional and behavioural problems). Demands are not true, they do not make sense and they do not help you get the thing you demand you must have (in fact, they make it less likely that you will). They are the rigid expression of a desire for something, and when it comes to the four thoughts that fuck you up, they sit at number one.

So, is there a way out of this madness? Can you fix that unhealthy thought? Can you correct the unhealthy demand and replace it with something more useful, helpful and rational? The answer is yes you can but, you'll have to wait for

Part Two to find out what that is because, when it comes to the thoughts that fuck you up, demands are only the tip of the disturbing iceberg. There are three other unhealthy thoughts that we need to take a look at first. Next one up is 'Doing a Drama'.

People who hold demands can also develop the tendency to blow things totally out of proportion . . .

Doing a Drama

There is nothing either good or bad but thinking makes it so.

William Shakespeare

Are words such as 'awful', 'nightmare' or 'catastrophe' a regular part of your vocabulary? What about 'terrible' and 'ruined'? If they are, it's time to ditch them now. Some people, when they have a demand for something, can 'awfulise' or catastrophise the problem. They take their problem, or the possibility of their demand not being met, and turn it into a total drama.

In the dictionary, awful has a specific meaning. It is used to describe something very bad or unpleasant: 'the weather was just awful' or 'don't eat there, the food is simply awful'. It's also used to emphasise the extent of something, especially if that something is also unpleasant or negative, as in, 'Oh dear, I seem to have made rather an awful fool of myself,' or, 'Did you hear what happened to poor Jane? It was so awful.'

However, in REBT, 'awful' has a very different meaning. It means you are making something far worse than it actually is. When you awfulise, things aren't just bad, they're

32

catastrophically bad – they're end-of-the-world bad, a 'nothing could be worse' kind of bad like your worst nightmare come true bad. In short, awful in REBT means 100 per cent bad.

Awfulising disturbs you because it is an extreme rating of how bad a given thing or situation is, or how bad it is that your demand has not been met. Some people awfulise in specific contexts, such as when they hold a particular demand about something, as in 'I must be on time for everything and it is awful when I am not,' for instance. If they are not in a situation that is triggering their demand, or if their demand is being met, they won't awfulise and they will naturally hold a much more realistic rating of the badness of any given situation.

Some people, however, awfulise in a more general way, or on a day-to-day basis. For them, everything is a nightmare, everything is terrible and everything is the end of the world. Perhaps you know people like this in your family, or in your social circle or among your colleagues at work? These are the sort of people who are always pointing out the worst case scenario in any given situation, the ones who happily point out everything that could go wrong with any idea you attempt to express, be it a business venture, a new purchase or a holiday. They are the ones you don't dare tell anything to for the fear that they'll just bring you down with their negativity. For life's awfulisers, life is indeed all doom and gloom.

Many of my clients over the years have admitted to being, or realised that they are, awfulisers, worst-case-scenario thinkers and all-round glass-half-empty kinds of people. Inside the therapy room, doing a drama is to be expected, but I also have the rather profound knack of being able to attract these people outside of the therapy room, in many different types of places but especially at bus stops. Why they pick me to talk to I do not know, it's not like I wear a T-shirt that says 'therapist' or anything, but it happened again only the other week.

A sudden heavy downpour caught me by surprise while out walking the dog and I ran to the cover of a nearby bus stop, where a little old lady was already waiting. I was pretty drenched. So was the dog. The lady looked at me, then tutted. 'Have you seen that weather?' she asked with a jerk of her head.

'Umm, yes?' I replied in a questioning fashion, just in case she wasn't referring to the clearly visible weather we both were witnessing from the relatively dry safety of the bus shelter.

'Terrible, isn't it?' she opined. 'Never seen anything like it.'

She didn't mean it in the dictionary definition sense of the word, as she wasn't just passing comment. She meant it in the fatalistic, REBT sense of the word. Her shoulders slumped as she said it, her voice was slow and down. The rain was truly troubling her. She sighed heavily.

'Err . . .' I said vaguely.

I decided not to mention yesterday's downpour, or last week's, or the one from the week before that, or any of the downpours from practically every week before that since time immemorial because, as you well know, this is the United Kingdom and that's just how the weather rolls here.

'Just terrible,' she repeated, and then lapsed into silence as we both waited out the rain with an uncomfortable black cloud that had nothing to do with the downpour hanging over the both of us. Awfulising: it can be a bit of a conversation killer.

For people like this, every downpour is awful. Every heatwave, every traffic jam, every missed appointment, every energy bill, and every single negative news story isn't just bad, it's the worst thing possible. When something goes wrong, it doesn't just go wrong – it gets ruined. They walk around in either a permanent fugue state or a state of high tension that can be infectious if you're not careful.

In and out of the therapy room, in specific contexts and with life in general, people can awfulise anything: not getting what they wanted, how people talk to them, how life has treated them and so on.

Words such as 'terrible' and 'awful' are part of everyday conversation, it is true. Some people can walk into a room and say, 'Look at that awful weather,' or, 'You look simply awful, John. Are you okay?' and then not disturb themselves (or anyone else for that matter). In REBT, the term 'awful' – and its relatives: terrible, nightmare, ruined, et al – only apply to those people who disturb themselves when they claim or believe that something is far worse than it actually is. These people are quick to anger, or depress themselves or are in a near-constant state of anxiety because of this extreme rating of the badness of the situation.

Take recreational drugs, for instance. Many people do. Some people take them because they are fun. They're not addicts, they are occasional recreational drug users. Whatever their drug of choice, they take it as part of a full and varied recreational social life that includes other people and other activities. Some people, however, take drugs to escape the pain and the misery of what they believe is the utter awfulness of their existence. They take drugs (or alcohol, or gambling, or sex and so on) to the exclusion of all else, or because they are convinced they have nothing else. These are the people at risk of becoming addicts. That's what believing something to be awful can do.

Our Friend, Disputing

And as with the demand, so to with the belief that something is awful: we need to dispute it. We hold it up to the bright illuminating light of rationality and ask, 'Hang on a minute. Is this belief true, does it actually make any sense and does it help me achieve my goal?'

We want to know if there is evidence to support that statement, either via observation or through experience. We want to highlight the sound reasoning behind this statement (or the lack thereof) and we want to see if it will help you to deal with things sensibly and realistically, or do the opposite. So, let's do that.

Consider the baldies (and I am one of them, remember). 'Being bald is awful,' many of them have claimed with conviction. 'My life is ruined.' And, as evidence that being bald was awful, they offer up examples such as: 'I don't like it', 'it makes me less of a man', 'I liked my hair', 'I won't get a partner', 'people will judge me', 'moulting hair blocks the sink', and so on.

Remember that in REBT 'awful' means 100 per cent bad, the worst thing that you can think of. For that to be true, it means you cannot think of worse. But you can. You can think of many things worse than being bald. No one is ill, no one is injured, no one has died, for a start. In short, the world did not end.

You are just bald. Every single thing that you can think of that is worse than being bald proves that being bald is not 'awful'.

However, the things that were proffered to me as evidence did highlight that being bald was bad in that (at the very least) none of those men who came to me liked it, and could ascertain negative consequences to their baldness. It might be bad; there might be negative consequences but, just because something is bad, it does not logically follow that the bad thing is an awful thing. They are, in fact, two different things. Bad exists on a scale of badness, from 0.01 per cent to 99.99 recurring per cent.[1] Imagine that anything and everything you can think of that is negative and bad can go on this scale, relative to every other bad thing that you place upon it. 'Awful' exists on a completely separate, non-existent, nonsensical scale of 100 per cent plus. If you don't like being bald, then it exists on your scale of badness, but it does not exist on the awful scale. Bad is one thing; but awful is another, completely different thing.

Believing that being bald is awful does not help you either. You are making it worse than it actually is. People who believe this make themselves miserable about the inevitable, can overlook people who actually find them attractive because they're too busy feeling unattractive, spend a fortune on treatments that don't actually work and more. What 'awful' does is blow everything out of proportion.

---

[1] Mathematicians and statisticians may disagree with this scale (and have done so, quite pointedly) but it's not meant to be scientifically accurate. It's an allegorical scale, a device used to make a point.

We have idioms in the English language that explain this process very clearly, such as 'making a mountain out of a molehill' and 'making a drama out of a crisis'. And that's what awfulising does, it makes the problem into the mountain and not the molehill; it gives any given crisis some added extra drama. In short (as one of my clients realised about himself only the other day), it turns you into a little bit of a drama queen.[2]

One of my friends finds it difficult talking to her mum on a regular basis because her mum is one such drama queen – an awfuliser of epic proportions; a non-stop litany of negativity; an endless rant against all the awful, terrible, downright rotten things that have happened to her, are happening to her and that probably will happen to her in the very near future. 'Say something nice,' my friend interjects forlornly whenever she can get a word in edgeways, in the vain hope that she can do something to break her mother's train of thought, or lift her mood a tad, but it rarely has the desired effect. My friend herself spends a lot of time worrying over the impact all that negativity has, not just on her mother's psyche, but also on her relationships with the other people around her and to the quality of her life in general.

Please note, when you seek to rationalise a drama out for yourself, when you begin to sift through the facts to find out if your particular 'awful' is true, or sensible or helpful (which it isn't); when you begin to think of all the things that are more bad than the thing you are thinking of please don't disturb

---

[2] Actually, a whole lot of a drama queen – an award-winning performance-level drama queen, even.

yourself further, as they are hardly likely to happen. Repeat: they are hardly likely to happen. All we are trying to do here is bring in balance and realise just how much you are blowing things out of proportion.

I've had so many clients make themselves anxious over the years, when the company they work for has sadly announced that they will have to make some redundancies. The people that made themselves anxious decided, without any facts to back this up, that one of the redundancies would definitely be theirs; that it must not happen and that it would be awful. Next, they are imagining all sorts: being fired, not finding another job, not being able to pay the bills or the mortgage, losing the house, being homeless, and so on. And all because of the beliefs they formulated in the face of a vague announcement.

Not everyone who holds a demand will awfulise when the demand is broken. You can hold a demand but not exhibit the tendency to rate the badness in an extreme way. Some people, however, do awfulise but are very much of the opinion that they don't. Just to be sure, it helps to think of the situation when you are at your most disturbed. When you are at your most angry, when you are at your most anxious, is it awful then? Think of 'in the moment' not 'after the moment'. Usually, after the moment means rationality has re-entered the room.

Others don't think they awfulise because they don't identify with the word itself. I had one client who was adamant that she did not awfulise or catastrophise, especially when it came to the problem we were working on, yet practically every week, at the start of her appointment she would want to schedule in a good few minutes to go off topic. This allowed her to vent about the dramas and crises that had arisen during the course of each particular week. The two phrases she used most often were, 'It was just terrible,' and, 'It was a total nightmare, I'm telling you.' However, she was definitely doing a drama here, because 'just terrible' and 'total nightmare, I'm telling you' meant 100 per cent bad.

Awfulising may not sound like a word, but it very much is a word. Many years ago, I worked in a particular environment that was very pressurised and deadline-driven. Every week something would go wrong with one of the many projects being worked on at any given time. Whenever something did go wrong, there was always a hard-core group of people who would huff and puff and scream out things such as, 'That's it, everything is ruined!' Or, 'This is completely fucked.'[3] Catastrophic was also used a lot to describe the various problems that arose and there they lurched, from week to week and from one seeming catastrophe to another. Except, nothing was completely fucked and nothing was ever ruined.

The awfulisers would step outside for a bit, to take a break, drink a coffee, smoke a cigarette, while inside work would continue as normal. All there ever was were problems, problems that were invariably resolved. It would have been nice if, on occasion, they could have dealt with a problem without claiming ruin or screaming catastrophe, but that was not their way.

---

[3] Which is what awfulising sounds like when it swears.

Nothing is ever awful and nothing is ever the end of the world – except for the end of the world. You can always think of something worse. Or be prompted into thinking of worse. And, if you can't, I can definitely think of worse, because I've had a lot of practice at it. And, if I can't (which is really rare) then someone else always can, because there are a lot of very imaginative people out there.[4]

Take my belief about crowds. When I demanded that other people must not get in my way, I also believed that it was awful when they did. But, that belief simply wasn't true. Even in the most crowded shopping mall, on the busiest shopping day of the year, with absolutely everybody bumping into me, tripping over me or tripping me up, I could still think of things that were worse; such as breaking a leg, being fired from a job, being dumped by the love of my life and so on. Sure, I didn't like crowds, I didn't like people that got in my way (and I didn't have to like them), but just because I didn't like them, just because 'other people getting in my way' sat on my scale of badness, it made no logical sense to conclude that it was awful. And, it certainly didn't help me. It turned me into a drama queen. And I was very, very dramatic about it. I'd shout, I'd swear, I'd shove and I would rally against the terrible unfairness of it all. I would go on about it for ages. I would growl like a bear. And it made me dread nice things, such as going to concerts and carnivals and festivals and fun days out.

I was also a horrible shopping companion, as many friends will attest.

---

[4] You sick, twisted puppies, you.

A Little Bit More About Badness

Some things are a little bit bad (being late, having people bump into you) and some things are fairly bad (such as being fired from a job you enjoy very much or being dumped by someone you are still totally in love with). Some things, however, are a whole lot bad; like really, really bad (such as domestic violence, being mugged or witnessing a traumatic incident). But, these things are still not 'awful' in REBT terms. No matter how bad something is, you can still always think of something worse. Even if it's only one thing, even if it's only slightly worse, or only theoretically worse, it still proves that the really bad thing is not an awful thing. This is not done to belittle or demean the incident, or what you went through, or how you feel. It is designed to help you move on, to put the incident behind you and get on with your life. Life can throw some pretty horrible things at you. But, no matter how horrible the horrible thing is, it is worse still to not be able to move on from it.

Challenging the awfulness of a distressing event sows the first seeds of doubt. It is the first step towards moving on, to reclaiming the life that you deserve, and you do owe it to yourself to move on. Whatever the horrible thing, you deserve to not be controlled or defined by that distressing event any more. Also, for something to be 100 per cent bad, it would also mean that you (or anyone else for that matter) are unable to show that any good came from it. But, even in the face of most traumatic of situations, you can usually evidence some good.

Take events such as earthquakes, tsunamis, forest fires and hurricanes.[5] When catastrophe strikes, there are always people to help, communities that rally, amazing tales of derring-do rescue and survival. Awful simply can't account for that, 100 per cent bad doesn't leave any room for these good things to happen.

There's a wonderful piece of advice from the American children's TV presenter, Fred Rogers (Mister Rogers), who once famously said, 'When I was a boy and I would see scary things in the news, my mother would say to me, "Look for the helpers. You will always find people who are helping."' In the midst of a disaster, you can always evidence some good.

And, for bald men everywhere, we can evidence Bruce Willis and Jason Statham, the money saved in haircuts, as well as opinion polls that find in favour of bald being sexy.

And, talking of good coming from bad. There's a video of a news clip doing the rounds on Facebook as I write this book. In the USA, one family lost their young daughter in an accident while on holiday. It's a horrible thing to happen to any family; it's an event no parent ever wants to go through. Yet sadly, and regrettably, many do.

In this particular instance, the family decided to donate their daughter's organs. Her organs saved many other lives, the lives of other children, to the immense gratitude of their respective parents. In the video, the girl's father cycled from

---

[5] Or typhoons, if you're anywhere near the Northwest Pacific; or cyclones, if you're in the vicinities of the South Pacific or Indian Ocean. 'Hurricane' only applies to the Atlantic and Northeast Pacific. In meteorology, location is everything.

Madison to Florida to raise awareness of (and support for) organ donation. Some 14,000 miles into the journey, in Baton Rouge, he meets the 21-year old man who received her heart. They hug and tearfully, the father listens with a stethoscope to his daughter's heart beating in the chest of this man.[6]

You cannot help but be moved by this; it's a lump-in-throat moment. While losing a loved one, especially if that loved one is your child, is very, very bad, here is something truly positive that came out of it.

Awful means you can't think of anything worse; awful means you can't evidence anything good. Awful is an unhealthy rating of the badness of your demand not being met or being broken. It often, but not always, goes hand in hand with the next unhealthy belief we are going to discuss.

The next thought that can fuck you up is officially called 'low frustration tolerance' and it's a rather rubbish rating of your ability to cope with all the challenging things that life can throw at you. It's an extreme assessment of your ability to deal with your demand being broken or with it not being met.

People who hold it don't believe they can cope with very much at all . . .

---

[6] No, you're crying.

The I Can't Copes

Problems are not the problem; coping is the problem.

Virginia Satir

This chapter is all about the 'I can't copes'. This unhealthy belief is also known as 'low frustration tolerance' (LFT), or 'I can't stand it'. AKA: 'I can't deal with that right now'.

Whereas awful is an extreme rating of how bad things are or, more specifically, how bad it is that a certain demand is not being met, low frustration tolerance is an extreme and unhealthy rating of your ability to cope with things: with emotions, with life situations, with other people and, more specifically, with your particular demand, similarly, not being met.

In terms of everyday language, it's when people say things such as 'I can't stand it' or 'I can't cope with this' or 'I can't handle this', and other such statements to that effect.

Take note, look around and listen. How many times this week have you heard 'I can't cope'. How many people around you have said, 'I can't cope with much more of this situation,' or, 'Oh dear god, not him/her/them. I can't stand much more of them.'

Just as with the other unhealthy beliefs, people often use low frustration tolerance in their everyday conversations. So, they say things such as, 'Isn't it wet? It's too wet. I can't cope with much more of this rain,' or, 'Have you met Julie's new boyfriend? I can't stand him.' But, they don't mean it in a disturbance-causing way; it is a figure of speech.

Some people, however, do mean it. Everything is intolerable, everything is unbearable, everything and everyone is way too much and everything is something they can't take much more of. And so they walk around in a permanent state of stress and exasperation or depression and more.

Many years ago, when I was travelling around, I worked briefly in a hotel pool bar in Turkish Cyprus. The manager placed me there as sales were low and he thought that having a non-Turkish, English-speaking person might be a draw. Sadly, he was right.

Every Monday, planeloads of English people would decant to the various hotels. When they made it to the one I was in and found me at the bar, they would say things such as, 'Oh, it's so nice to hear a familiar voice.'[1]

As I was there at the end of the year, they were also happy to tell me how cold it was back home. They would tell me all about the snow, the ice and the rain, how unbearable it all was, and just how happy they all were to be far away from it all; to be somewhere that was nice and sunny. This lasted for all of four or five days. And then low frustration tolerance would kick in.

---

[1] Despite having been there for all of five minutes or so.

'Isn't it hot?' the self-same people would say. 'It's too hot. I can't cope with much more of this heat. Any more of this and I'm going to die. I can't wait to get back home.'

They may or may not have been disturbing themselves, but they were putting a slight crimp in my travelling experience.

But when people exhibit low frustration tolerance, they will disturb themselves. They will experience unhealthy negative emotions and they will behave in self-defeating ways.

People who have a hefty dose of the 'I can't copes' have a profound inability to tolerate unpleasant feelings or difficult emotions or adverse situations and events. People with LFT want things the way they want them to be and will decide that things are simply intolerable if not; that any and all frustrations have to be resolved quickly and easily and will disturb themselves whenever and wherever they are not. People who believe they can't cope also have a tendency to avoid the frustrating thing, which only leads to increased frustration, which leads to more avoidance. Avoidance becomes an unhealthy coping strategy in the face of said frustration. Other unhealthy coping strategies can creep in too.

People who feel they can't cope may attempt to medicate their frustrations with alcohol, with drugs (both prescription and recreational) and, even, with food.

I've had plenty of people present to my clinic with what they thought were alcohol or drug problems, or an unhealthy relationship with food, when, actually the drug or the drink or the food was a crutch, a way of coping with the thing they felt they couldn't cope with.

I had one memorable client who came to me because she thought she was an alcoholic, so did her friends and so too did her partner, who had delivered an ultimatum that facilitated the call to me. But, while she did have a drink problem, drink was not *the* problem. She was not an alcoholic, but she was a bit of a control freak and, because of it, a very nervous traveller.

She didn't like any and all situations that were not under her control. Such situations took her way out of her comfort zone and, to compensate, she drank. This problem with control acutely manifested itself in transport. She didn't like flying, she didn't like trains and she didn't like travelling on coaches because she wasn't in the driving seat, or the pilot's seat. Handing control over to someone else really was not her cup of tea. So she drank vodka instead.

She could drive, but she couldn't afford to run a car, hence the reliance on other modes of transport. She sat through most journeys in a heightened state of anxiety. So, to cope with her anxiety, she drank. Copiously. She flew quite often for work and travelled a fair bit on trains and by coach to see various family members and, in particular, her partner. And, because she generally arrived at any and all destinations in quite the state of inebriation, her friends, family and partner assumed she had a drink problem. Which she then also assumed.

But, when we worked on her beliefs about control, when we worked on her anxiety about control (of which low frustration tolerance played a very large part) and, as she got that anxiety under her control, her drinking patterns naturally returned to normal. As she no longer needed booze to help her deal with transport, she returned to what she had been before this problem started – a social drinker.

There are many people, some of whom may be reading this, who are medicating themselves with Xanax and beta-blockers and such-like because they believe they cannot cope with their anxiety. There will be people reading this who feel so unable to cope with the demands of the day that, at the end of the day, they promise themselves a glass of wine, but end up downing the whole bottle, or who promise themselves just the one biscuit, but then devour the whole packet.

There are people reading this who self-harm because they believe they can't cope with their emotions, or the intensity of their emotions or, even, life in general.

In extreme situations, people who believe they can't cope with their emotions or the state of their lives, may attempt to end that life. This ultimate act of avoidance becomes the only coping strategy they believe they have left. Suicide is devastating for all concerned, as are the unhealthy beliefs behind it.

I was talking to a teacher friend of mine while writing this book, and he reckons that LFT lies behind a lot of his pupils' emotional and behavioural problems. He tells me his pupils say, 'I can't cope,' and, 'I can't stand it,' several times a day.

They can't cope with the amount of homework; they can't cope with the pressures of needing to get good grades, or having got bad grades; or the pressures of exams; or the need to be popular, or the misery of being unpopular; or social media; or bullying (online or otherwise); or their emotions or, basically, life in general.

It's quite possible that this problem is then carried forward from schools and into universities as practically every single university's counselling department is swamped. It's full of people who say they cannot cope with the pressures of life and study at said university.

But low frustration tolerance does more than just weaken our resolve and our fortitude.

Human beings are programmed for comfort. We seek it out and we favour it. We will seek instant gratification to ward off boredom; we will eat the doughnut, despite wanting to be beach-body ready by July; we will take the drug we don't want to, rather than deal with the difficulty of saying no. In short, we sacrifice our long-term goals in favour of a short-term gain. And so, an attack of the 'I can't copes' can turn us into hedonists, thrill-seekers and creatures of the moment.

Neuroscience has a lot to say about why we humans prefer the easy way out. There's no definitive answer as yet, but most agree that the impulse is hardwired. Hardwired, however, does not mean 'impossible to change', it just means 'difficult to change'.

Believing you can't cope is a huge contributor to stress, so much so that it's pretty much built into any definition of stress. However, there are actually two types of stress: good stress and bad stress.

Good stress is known as 'eustress'. Think of the excitement of getting married, or the deadline on a major project you are enjoying, or a rollercoaster ride.[2]

Bad stress is known as 'distress', but this has simply been reduced to the word 'stress' over time.

---

[2] If you enjoy rollercoaster rides that is; if you don't and you're on one, you will experience bad stress. And, quite possibly, vomit.

In the UK, work stress is the number one cause of staff sickness and absenteeism. The Health and Safety Executive (HSE) formal definition of work-related stress is 'the adverse reaction people have to excessive pressures or other types of demand placed on them at work'. Simply put, if you feel that you can cope with the pressure, you will feel the good type of stress but, if you feel that you can't cope, you will experience the bad kind of stress.

That HSE definition applies not just to work but to practically any and all situations you can think about: study, life, people, income, status, you name it – anywhere you feel a pressure, anyone you feel is applying a pressure, either real or imagined.

Stress is a catch-all term and it can lead to anger-management issues, to depression, to anxiety, to addictions and more. I had one client who came to see me because she was stressed. When I asked her what she got stressed about, she said, 'Everything.' When we touched upon LFT, when I introduced it as a concept but hadn't actually started working on it as part of a specific demand, she had the realisation that she was pretty much intolerant of, well, nearly everything and everyone, but most importantly, intolerant of deadlines and the people who didn't make the deadlines, or do the work the way she wanted it done. When things were not going the way she wanted them to, she felt pressure. A pressure that she found intolerable, that she just could not deal with. She realised that, more often than not, to relieve that pressure, she used the line, 'Just get it fucking done, will you?' only not like a statement, or an edict, and not even like a weapon to inflict damage, but more like a shield or a talisman. It became an unhealthy way of relieving the pressure she felt. This was at work.

She was equally stressed at home but this was more because, even though she wanted to say, 'Just get it fucking done, will you?' she couldn't, because this was her family she was dealing with not her employees. Either way, she realised pretty quickly that she lived a life of near-constant frustration. She realised that her mantra meant 'I can't cope'. It meant she couldn't cope with excuses, or trusting people to meet dead-lines, or meeting her exacting standards, that she couldn't cope with people who asked too many questions rather than get on with it, or the people who didn't do it the way she would do it.

In REBT, there are four types of 'I can't cope'. There is:

- Emotional intolerance – where you can't deal with emotional distress
- Entitlement intolerance – where you can't stand unfairness or frustrated gratification
- Discomfort intolerance – where you can't deal with difficulties or hassles
- Achievement intolerance – where you can't deal with not achieving your goals

People believe they can't cope with work; that they can't stand certain people; that they can't deal with being thwarted; that they can't handle certain situations and more. And yes, there are some people who believe they can't cope with not being on time for everything. There's even a low-level kissing cousin to LFT, known as 'I can't be bothered' or 'I can't be arsed'. Also, in my experience, the word 'unbelievable' can sometimes be an 'I can't cope' in disguise.

Kissing Cousins to the I Can't Copes

If you are an arch procrastinator, low frustration tolerance (LFT) is a very likely culprit. Sometimes, you're putting off the thing you know you need to do because you've had an attack of the 'I can't copes'. That is, you genuinely feel that you can't deal with the thing but, more often, it's more stealthy than that, it's your mind simply telling you that you can't be bothered to do it right now.

Going back to the guy I mentioned in the introduction, the one who wanted to know why he didn't always clean the fish tank out on time. Although the tutor at the time was right, and no one would pay a therapist good money to work on this as a problem, the answer was easy. The answer was that he held an unhealthy belief, and that belief was 'I can't be arsed'. And so, more often than not, he put off cleaning the fish tank until it was really, really dirty, or when the very lives of his fish were imperilled by filth.

Avoiding difficult situations can prevent us from dealing with problems constructively, and even prevent us from dealing with them at all: ending a relationship, quitting your job and so on. But, 'I can't be bothered' will prevent you from enacting a healthy lifestyle, or tackling anything you perceive as boring, or difficult and demanding of your time, or that will simply take more effort than you feel willing to give.

When working in London I used to see this year in and year out with students on higher education courses who had allowed lengthy essays, such as dissertations and theses, to pile up. A thesis is boring (unless you really like doing them). It involves being inside, sat at a desk, reading dull, dry books and research articles. They're usually set with an end of summer deadline; which means working through both spring and summer. But these months are fun months. Winter has passed, life is in bloom, the days lengthen and there is always fun to be had. A nice night out here; or a naughty night in there, who wouldn't want some of that after a long and gruelling winter? Reading, research and writing, by contrast, well that's just boring and tedious. It requires effort, it requires sacrifice, but you can't be bothered. You promise yourself that you will do it, but then the phone rings and someone fun with something fun to do comes calling and so you go out, promising to do it tomorrow, or at the weekend; or next week, at the very latest. Or, you'd sit down to do it sometimes but then you'd get bored and go and do something else, something you kid yourself is constructive, but isn't: something simple, like cleaning the kitchen or tidying your room. Sure, the house is now spotless, but the dissertation still needs to be done and, all of a sudden the deadline is looming, staring you right in the face and there you are, sitting in my chair, wailing, 'I don't know why I always do this.'

Low frustration tolerance is why.

The word 'unbelievable', in my experience, can also be a low frustration tolerance belief. I have worked with many people that way. Sometimes, something really, really horrible or shocking happens, or someone does something really, really unthinkable. And people get stuck; they get hooked on 'unbelievable'. They can't believe it. They say things such as, 'I can't believe he did that,' or, 'I can't believe that happened, I just can't.' This is just another way of saying, 'I cannot cope with this knowledge.'

I can't cope, I can't stand it, I can't deal with that right now, I can't be arsed, I can't be bothered and it's unbelievable. They are all LFT beliefs. They will disturb you, they will lead to very poor emotional and behavioural outcomes, and they will not help you achieve your goals.

A Simple Hack

Before we move on to disputing low frustration tolerance. I want to talk to you about flipping your buts. And, by but, I mean the word 'but' and not your posterior.[3] It's not an REBT technique per se but, if you're suffering from low-level low frustration tolerance, it can be surprisingly effective.

Let's say that you have joined a gym, you want to get fit and you want to get toned but, every night, you come home from work and you say, 'Well, I do want to go to the gym, *but* I'm just too tired.' So, you don't go. Or, you're on a diet, but it's always someone's birthday or anniversary at work so someone is

---

[3] I'm really, really, not asking you to twerk.

always bringing in cake or chocolates, or both. 'Well, I know I want to lose a few pounds, *but* I really like the look of that cake,' you say, and you eat the cake. Every time. The problem is the 'but' and what follows it. In the first instance, your focus isn't on the gym, it's on feeling tired, so you don't go to the gym; and, in the second instance, your focus isn't on losing a few pounds, it's on the cake. So, you eat it.

But, what if you came home from work and said, 'Well, I know I'm tired, but I really want to go to the gym.' What would happen then? What if someone at work was passing around another plump and juicy-looking piece of birthday cake and you said, 'Well, I know I like the look of that cake, but I really want to lose a few pounds.' What would you do now?

Chances are, you would go to the gym and you would say a simple, but definitive, 'no' to the cake because you've flipped your 'buts' and placed the focus of that sentence on the thing you really want.

One client of mine, after I had taught him the basics of REBT and the differences between a demand and a preference, came back with a startling revelation. Doughnuts, chocolates and biscuits were office favourites where he worked and saying no to all three things was his goal. He noticed that the next time someone came in with a box of doughnuts, every single person who said, 'Oh, I really shouldn't, but they do look lovely,' had one (or more) of the doughnuts; but the one person who said, 'Mmm, I'd like one, but I'm watching my figure,' said no and didn't take any.

Flip your buts this week. I'm not promising anything, but you never know what you may be able to accomplish.

Our Friend, Disputing

And, on to disputing because, like the unhealthy beliefs before them, none of your 'I can't copes' are true, none of them make sense and none of them help you.

As a quick question, I just want to ask: are you dead? Have you ceased to be? Is it that you are reading this from beyond the grave? Of course the answer is a resounding 'no'. If it isn't, then I am in the wrong job, and I should have become a professional medium years ago. If you are alive, then it simply cannot be true that you cannot stand or cope with the thing you say you cannot stand or cope with. Just think about what the words 'I can't stand it' mean. If you literally could not stand something, you would be dead; it would end you, you would cease to be.

For those of you that don't believe me, I'm going to talk about lobsters. Have you ever eaten lobster? Do you know how one is typically cooked? It is picked up alive and plopped in a pot of boiling hot water. The process kills it, because a lobster cannot stand being boiled in water. And nor could you for that matter. If we tried to serve you up as Larry, Laura or Leal Thermidor, while I can't say if you'd be as succulent as the lobster, I do know you would not be able to stand being boiled in water. You would die. That is what 'I can't stand it' literally means. You are the proof that negates the 'I can't copes'. Living, breathing, walking, talking you proves that 'I can't stand it' is not true. So, just think of all the things you say you cannot stand, and then disprove them by remembering that you are alive. You have stood them, and you will continue to stand them.

*

Let's take the belief 'I can't stand not being on time'. This is not true. Despite the delay, you did not die and you got there in the end. Sure, you might have missed the meeting or you might have had to work late and these things might make your day difficult. But, difficult doesn't kill you.

I'm delayed often on a Thursday as I take the train to London and back, but my life goes on. I endure.[4] Now, maybe you're not coping with things as well as you would like. It happens. We don't always cope as well as we would want. If you're angry, or anxious or depressed, if you're using alcohol or Xanax as a coping strategy, then it is safe to assume that you are not dealing with things very well, that you find them difficult, challenging and frustrating. However, despite finding something difficult, it logically follows that you can stand it, that you can bear it, that you can cope.

Going back to timekeeping. It's quite rational to say, 'I pride myself on my punctuality, so not being on time for everything is a challenge for me,' or, 'Not being on time for everything can put a severe kink in my day.' But, it doesn't make any sense to say, 'I can't stand being on time because I don't like it.' One is rational (I find this thing difficult) and the other is not (therefore it is unbearable); they're saying two different things, therefore one cannot logically be concluded from the other. If the statement did make sense, then logically we'd have to apply that rule to all human beings. Where would we be if human beings could not tolerate delay? We would not be here, we would be extinct; we'd still be in the ocean, eyeing the land and thinking, 'I don't like the look of that.' Human

---

[4] Not only as in 'remain in existence' but also as in 'suffer patiently'.

58

beings tolerate adversity on a daily basis; it's how we grow and develop, it is how we become resilient.

Believing that you cannot cope, that you cannot stand something, certainly does not help you. It leads to psychological disturbance, it strips you of your resilience, it disempowers you, makes you weak, prevents you from using rational coping strategies (such as 'getting on with it' or 'problem solving') and allows unhealthy coping strategies to creep in (such as avoidance and delay, or alcohol and drugs). And, in extreme circumstances, it can cause you to think about, plan and even execute a suicide attempt.

People who believe they can't stand it when they are not on time for everything tend to arrive ridiculously early for their appointments. One of my clients, who did indeed have a bit of a thing for punctuality, always arrived so early for her appointments with me that she had plenty of time to kill. So she killed it with several cups of coffee in a nearby coffee shop. In our sessions, she was often very jittery and frequently in need of toilet breaks.

If you are reading this book then, despite every phrase you have uttered along the lines of 'I can't cope with this', you have actually survived. You have survived every single difficulty and challenge you have so far faced. That's a 100 per cent success rate. How cool is that?

As far as I know, every one of those holidaymakers I met in the hotel made it home alive and, in all likelihood, went on to book future sunny holidays that they then said they couldn't cope with nary five days into their trip.

So, get rid of the 'I Can't Copes'. Phrases such as this have no place in your vocabulary, or in your mindset or as part of your belief system. Unless, that is, you are applying it to something that would actually kill you.[5]

Let's go back to my belief about crowds. Did I believe that people getting in my way was intolerable, that they were something I could not cope with? Totally. 'I can't stand it when other people get in my way,' I said. In fact, I probably held this belief more than any other. To me, crowds were absolutely unbearable. This was simply not true though – I had not died as a result of someone getting in my way. None of the people who had bumped into me, or stumbled over me or come to a dead stop right in front of me had ever been the cause of my demise. I found crowded places full of people milling around and getting in my way difficult to deal with for sure, but just because I found it a challenge it did not make any sense to conclude that it was unbearable. If it did make sense then, when taken to a logical conclusion, people getting in the way would be pretty much an extinction-level event.

And it most certainly did not help me to believe this drama. Because of this belief I mostly avoided crowded places, even the enjoyable ones that I really wanted to go to. If I did find myself in a crowded place, or made it out to a place I wanted to enjoy, then my fuse became a very short fuse indeed. And, it often led to tears and screams of horror.[6]

Disputing also applies to those kissing cousins, 'I can't be bothered' and 'I can't believe it'. 'I can't be bothered' is not true. If you have managed to bother with something you could not be bothered with before (be it going to the gym,

---

[5] Boiling water, *et al*.

[6] Not all of them mine.

completing that project or thesis or what have you) then you have proof that I can't be bothered is not true. Saying something is unbelievable is also not true. It doesn't matter how horrible or shocking it is, it happened. If it hadn't happened, you wouldn't be in a state of disbelief.

Saying something is boring, or that you find it hard to motivate yourself is rational; saying you can't be bothered just because you find it hard to bother or be motivated is not rational, therefore one does not logically flow from the other. Similarly, just because you find something very difficult to get your head around, it does not logically follow that it is unbelievable. They are two different concepts and one does not logically flow from the other.

Believing 'I can't be bothered' certainly does not help you: it leads to procrastination, to putting off the things you need to do. 'I can't believe it' doesn't help you either. It keeps you stuck in a state of shock and disbelief instead. People who believe 'I can't believe it' find it very difficult to move on from the things they say they can't believe.

So, if you're dealing with an attack of the 'I can't copes' – also known as 'I can't stand it' or low frustration tolerance and sometimes expressed as 'I can't be bothered' or 'I can't believe it' – then just remember that it's not true, it does not make sense and it does not help you.

And with that, we can move on to our final unhealthy belief, the fourth thought that fucks you up, and the one that is probably the most persistent, insidious and prevalent of all. The people who hold it can feel really, really shit about both themselves and other people. And that's not fun at all . . .

Pejorative Put-Downs

No one can make you feel inferior without your consent.

Eleanor Roosevelt

The fourth and final thought that can really, really fuck you up – number four in our queasy quartet of unhealthy beliefs that disturb, disrupt and generally deliver poor psychological results – can actually veer off into any one of three directions.

When people don't get what they demand they 'must' have, when things go wrong, or when life seems stacked against them, they can develop the tendency to 1) put themselves down; or they can 2) put other people down, or they can even 3) put world conditions down.

In REBT, putting yourself down is known as self-damning. People who do this tend to see themselves as stupid, useless, worthless, no-good failures (or they call themselves certain derogatory swear word terms). Putting other people down is known as 'other-damning', and it's where you tend to see other people as stupid, useless, worthless, no-good failures (or you apply certain derogatory swear word terms to them as opposed to yourself).

People can also apply these terms to the world in total (as in 'the world is useless' or 'life is no good'); or to certain life conditions, such as work (boring) or relationships (mine totally sucks). This is known as 'world-damning'. And again, you can label these things with negative words and phrases.

Similarly to I can't copes, we don't always mean these statements. Conversationally, people say things such as, 'Oh my god, I'm such a twat,' or 'You're such an idiot,' and they don't really mean it, or they don't disturb themselves by saying it or are even saying it in a jovial, friendly and inclusive way.[1]

But we can really mean it: when we are disturbed and dysfunctional; when we are angry, anxious or depressed; when we hold unhealthy demands. In those moments, we do. The terms become global definitions, all-encompassing descriptors, and we become unable to see ourselves, others or certain things any other way. Here, the put-down isn't an innocent comment or a jovial piece of banter; it has become an all-defining characteristic.

For some people, this self-doubt is mild: they feel like a bit of a failure, so they assume that they are a failure. They feel a little stupid compared to other people, so they conclude that they are stupid. But, for others, it's much, much deeper; it's total and utter self-loathing. It's self-hatred on an enormous scale. They see themselves as abject failures – utterly worthless, useless, fat, ugly, stupid, no-good write-offs.

People like this can not only hate themselves, but they can also depress themselves, and feel guilty for being the inferior,

---

[1] 'You twat' is, more often than not, a term of endearment here in the UK.

worthless nothings that they have decided they are. In short, their self-esteem is shot to shit. What could anyone possibly have done to hate themselves so much?

One of the most common problems that people present with when they seek out the services of a therapist or coun-sellor (either directly, or as part-and-parcel of their other problems) is that of self-esteem issues, or confidence. I've lost count of the amount of times people have contacted me because they have issues such as these either directly or indirectly. And the problem lies within the very term itself: self-esteem.

To esteem something is to respect, admire, regard, deem, value, judge and rate that thing. The word itself comes from the Latin 'aestimare' (to estimate). So, with self-esteem, you are, quite literally, rating or valuing yourself. You are estimat-ing yourself.

Some people over-estimate themselves. 'Look at me,' they say, 'I'm fantastic!') But, let's face it, people who over-estimate themselves rarely, if ever, come to therapy. In all my years of practice, I've never had someone come to see me saying, 'Can you help me please? I over-estimate myself, I feel like I am totally awesome and I need you to help bring me down a peg or two.'[2]

No, most people, especially the ones coming to therapy, and sadly, many more who don't, tend to under-estimate themselves. Some downright denigrate themselves based on, well, not much in particular at all.

---

[2] Although, I bet you know a few people you'd like to put forward for therapy to work on this exact thing.

Basing your confidence on how you estimate yourself is a very dangerous game indeed.

'Self-esteem is the greatest sickness known to man or woman,' said Albert Ellis. 'Because it is conditional.' The more things you've got going for you, the more success you can evidence and the more trappings you can display, then the higher your confidence levels get. However, the more you get wrong; the more you cock it up and the more failures you can show, then the lower your confidence levels sink.

The trouble is we get it right and wrong and we succeed and we fail on an almost daily basis so, when you play self-esteem's rating game, your confidence is like a yo-yo. It's going up one minute and down the next, all depending on what you have and have not achieved. Up and down and up and down and on and on. Exhausting isn't it?

Also, when it comes to confidence issues, most of us are rating ourselves in the overwhelmingly negative. So when things get really bad, the yo-yo stays stuck in 'down'. When things go wrong, people give themselves a global rating: failing a driving test means you are a complete failure; getting a few things wrong means you are totally useless; tuck a couple of failed relationships under your belt and suddenly you're a total love loser; sink into depression and you end up believing you're completely worthless.

It's easy to do this, it's easy to play the rating game and come up wanting. We live in a world that plays the rating game – at school, at work, on the television, in magazines, almost everywhere. We're taught to compete, to be better than, to constantly improve, that our life is not worth living if we're not living our best possible life.

And, sadly, some people have family or friends, or end up in relationships with people, who tell them that they are rubbish, bit by bit, slowly and over time, until it's the only thing they can believe about themselves.

It's easy to look around and see everybody else seem to be doing so much better than you and so you come up wanting. If you feel like a failure, then it must be so: you are a failure, you suck. If the other person keeps being rude to you, then they must be a total arse, they are an idiot, they suck; if you're not satisfied in your job, then the job is completely pointless and has no redeeming features, it too sucks.

Going back to the analogy about timekeeping, someone could be sitting on a delayed train believing 'I must be on time for everything, it's all my fault that I'm not, I'm so stupid' (and make themselves anxious). Someone else could be sitting on the same train believing 'I must be on time for everything, it's all the manager's fault that I'm not, he's such an idiot' (and get angry with the on-board services manager on duty at the time). Meanwhile, someone else could be sitting on that train believing 'I must be on time for everything, it's the train operating company's fault that I am not, this franchise is not fit for purpose' (and still get angry in a more generalised way).[3]

But, are things as they appear? Let's say it is actually your fault that you are late – is that all there is to you? Are you nothing but the failure of being late on this occasion? If it is actually the fault of the manager, or the driver or the network,

---

[3] But the on-board services manager may still cop it; empathise with the on-board services manager, be nice to them.

or all three combined. Is that all there is to them? It's all rather one-dimensional, isn't it?

Nothing is one-dimensional (except in maths) and no one is one-dimensional. It's all much more complicated than that. As the retired clinical psychologist and author Dr Paul Hauck once put it, the self is 'every conceivable thing about you that can be rated'.[4]

And he meant everything. So, that definition includes your thoughts, feelings, behaviours and skills (or lack thereof), as well as your achievements, failings, body parts and more – absolutely everything about you from birth until death, everything you have ever done and ever will do going forwards from now.

And when you look at it like that, rating yourself totally negatively based on one or two undesirable attributes really doesn't do 'you' any justice at all, does it?

How old are you right now? Are you 22, 37 or 84? It doesn't matter how old you are, what I want to know is: can you sit there and rate every single thing about you so far? Can you forward project and rate every conceivable thing going forwards? Can you grab a piece of paper and put down a 'tick' for every positive attribute and a 'cross' for every negative one? You could try but that would be an endeavour far larger than even the Human Genome Project.[5]

---

[4] And he said it in many places, including *Overcoming the Rating Game: Beyond Self-Love, Beyond Self Esteem*.

[5] The Human Genome Project ran from 1990 to 2003 and mapped and identified every single one of the several thousand or so genes present in human DNA. This could help eradicate disease and make medicine more effective (good) but could also be weaponised and even create 'designer' humans (bad).

If you can evidence any one positive in your life, any successes at all, then it simply is not true that you are a total failure. Just because you have failed your test, it makes no sense to judge yourself totally (as a loser). Just because you failed in one or two relationships, it really does not help you to say that you are totally worthless (instead it leaves you feeling unlovable). You only need one tick to prove the point – just one 'tick' in the picture of you would prove that you are not a failure, or stupid or useless. But, you have more than one tick. Each and every tick is a piece of proof.

And we can back this up with pure, objective rationality. We can back this up by disputing, by asking if these put-down beliefs are true, whether or not they make sense and whether or not they help you. (Big hint: they do not.)

Self-damning is not true, it can't be true. If you wrote down a list of your skills, your accomplishments, your qualifications (either academic or vocational or from the school of life), the things you are proud of, the things you have done well or got right, what would that list include? If you put down a series of 'ticks' to represent your successes, how many would there be and what would they represent?

Feel free to write that list down now if you have a pen and pad handy; just write down a few things that take in the above. Or simply formulate a brief list in your head: tick after tick after tick.

The items on that list are facts, they are evidence; each tick is a piece of proof that proves that you cannot be a failure, that you cannot be useless or worthless, or a complete fuck-up. If you were, would there be any ticks or items on this list at all? The answer is no and yet, ticks there are, many of them in fact.

Despite what your feelings are telling you, you have evidence here against this belief, evidence that is staring you right in the face. Now, it may be that your confidence is so low that you are struggling to come up with anything much at all. It doesn't matter. Even if you can only come up with one or two things, then this is enough at this point to prove you are not a total failure, that you are not totally stupid.

Take me for instance, I have self-damned in the past. I have felt like an abject failure because I believed in my heart that I was. I've believed that I wasn't good enough and that my past mistakes had rendered me useless, and yet I've got several diplomas and two degrees under my belt. I landed a job at a prestigious magazine on graduating from university after studying journalism, I built a successful therapy practice up from scratch. I love using REBT and hypnotherapy to help people out of their personal ruts. I'm kind to people and animals; I love my dog and I always feed my friend's fish when they're away on holiday. These are 'ticks' in a picture of me, positive attributes in that picture. How could I be a total failure if I can prove such things? What about you? What have you evidenced as you read this?

Many years ago I had a client come to see me to help him with his addiction to cannabis. He was such the consummate stoner that his boyfriend had left him and he'd lost his job. He was in such a bad way that even his dealer had cut him off and told him he needed help, which is why he had contacted me.

He saw himself as an abject failure, a total loser. When I tried to get him to come up with things he was good at, some positive attributes in the picture of him, he was unable to. He was so depressed at what had happened that he couldn't find one positive thing to say about himself. 'How can I?' he said bleakly. 'I'm so useless even my drug dealer refuses to see me.'

After a while, I said, 'I bet I know something you're good at.' He eyed me suspiciously.

'In fact,' I ventured, 'I bet I know something you're brilliant at.'

'What?' He asked defensively. 'You don't even know me.'

'I bet you roll the best joints,' I said. 'I bet you can roll one in a force 10 gale, with your eyes closed.'

'I can't believe you just said that,' he said.

It was a risky move but there, I'd said it. 'I bet it's true though, or close enough to the truth,' I replied.

'Well, yes,' he said. 'But there's more to me than that.' And then, with a bit more coaxing, he started talking about all the things he was good at before he become such a stoner. We all make mistakes, but those mistakes don't erase past accomplishments, or prevent future successes.

Saying you are a failure, or that you are stupid, or rubbish or what-have-you does not make sense. Yes, there are things in life you have failed at. You have made mistakes and got things wrong. There are things in this world that you are just no good at. You can draw up a list of these things too, if you want.

However, you can rate individual aspects of yourself. For instance, I'm no good at DIY or maths. I've made mistakes (some of them really big; like, really, really big; like let's just sweep them under the carpet and forget about them big). I also lost the job on that prestigious magazine; I've accidentally hurt people, failed job interviews, and forgotten who people are. I can be bossy; I've let people down. I could go on.

These are crosses in the same picture of me, negative aspects that I possess. We all have them.

Now, if I said to you, 'I have failed my driving test, therefore I am a failure,' would you tell me I was making sense? I'm hoping the answer is no. But, what if I said, 'Actually that was a bit of a fib, I've actually failed my driving test a hundred times now, so that must mean I am a failure.' Would you tell me I was making sense because of it? Hopefully, your answer is still no. So, what answer would make sense?

Maybe I have a poor relationship with my driving instructor. Change the instructor, and I change the outcome. Or, maybe, I have an exam anxiety issue. Deal with that issue in REBT, get my anxiety under control and I can change the outcome. Or, maybe, I just need to accept that I am no good at driving. Maybe I should never be allowed behind the wheel of a car. Maybe I need to give up on my goal of being a taxi driver. But, here's the clincher: being no good at driving does not make me no good as a person. Failing at something, or even a few things, does not make me a complete failure. One does not logically flow from the other.

It certainly doesn't help you to put yourself down. It will depress you; it will make you anxious; it will eat away at your faith in yourself until you have none; it will make you compare yourself to others and always, always come up short. In fact, it does nothing but disturb you.

So, self-damning is not true, does not make sense and does not help you. But, what about damning other people? Well, other people are not useless, or stupid, or worthless, or completely rotten <insert expletive of choice here>.

71

As it is with you, so too is it with them. You may not know them well, you may not know them at all, but they all have ticks in the picture of them as well. They all have positive aspects and such-like. They have skills and qualifications (either academic or vocational or school of life), they have strengths and things they are good at. They have people who love them and they probably do nice things for people. Maybe not for you, not always, but they do. If you can evidence so much as one single, solitary positive aspect about another human being then they cannot be that thing you believe them to be: it's simply not true.

Again, like you, they have failings, weakness and bad points. They've made mistakes. Maybe they've made mistakes with you, which is why you are putting them down in the first place. But, a failing does not make them a complete failure; a mistake (or two, or several) does not make them a complete write-off. It makes no sense to define a person in their entirety based on one, two or a few negative attributes.

And it does not help you. This isn't about them. This is about you. Other-damning disturbs you; it makes you angry; it makes you demonise the other. You carry grudges. It can even make you hate, hurt and disparage the people that you profess to love.

There's a simple exercise that some therapy groups engage in, especially anger-management groups. The therapist brings in a big bowl of stones – large ones – and asks the group members to pick up a stone for every grudge they are holding. Every. Single. One. They are then asked to carry those stones around in their pockets for a whole week. What do you think that feels like? Heavy, don't you think? Burdensome? That is what putting other people down does to you. What do you think it feels like to pop the stones back in the bowl at the end of the exercise? What would it feel like if you stopped putting other people down right now, today?

And, finally, on to world-damning. Firstly, the world is not completely shit. It may feel like it sometimes, especially when you read or listen to the news. But, it isn't. Right now, think of three things you like about the world. They could be ice cream, rainbows, elephants or anything. The same goes for your job – your job is not completely shit, even if you dislike it intensely right now. Think of three things you like about your job, it could be the fact that it pays for stuff or that your colleagues are nice, or, simply that it's near home.

So, if you can demonstrate positive things about such things, then those things can't be as useless, rubbish or shit as you say they are. The world, your job and life conditions do contain negatives. But, just because they contain negatives, it makes no sense to completely write them off, to judge them as completely negative because of it.

And again, put-downs about the world or life conditions will not help you. You will despair over the world, or your job; you will become disturbed and dysfunctional but, in all likelihood, you won't do anything about it.

Take timekeeping. 'I must be on time for everything,' you say, 'and it's all my fault if I'm not, I'm such an idiot.' Or you might say that the manager is an idiot or claim that the network is not fit for purpose.

But, if you're late, you're late. It might be your responsibility and it might not but, it's simply not true to say you are an idiot because of it; it's not true to say the manager is an idiot (he holds down his job for a start) and it's not true that the rail operator is a write-off as you can evidence good things about them. Even if it is your fault that you were late, even if you did an idiotic thing, it still makes no sense to say you are a complete idiot just because you did something silly. 'That was silly' and 'I'm an idiot' are two different things. One does not logically flow from the other.

It's the same thing with the manager. And, it's the same again with the train operating company. And none of these beliefs help you. You are still on a delayed train, only you're angry with yourself, or you're shouting at the manager or you're storming off the train in a huff.

Back to my belief about crowds: Was I damning? You bet I was, but I wasn't self-damning – as I was fine, I was righteous and I wasn't the one getting in my way. Neither were my put-downs of the 'world'. No, my put-downs were about other people. Other people were complete idiots to me. Not just the ones that actually got in my way, but all of them. Because each and every individual in a crowded situation was eyed by me with suspicion because they all had the potential to either become the person that got in my way, or be the cause of someone else getting in my way; ergo, all of them were total pillocks.[6]

This is of course not true. It's true I did not know them but, on an observational level, they could, at the very least, dress themselves, perambulate and navigate trains, stations, ticket

---

[6] Except on the very (and I want to make this perfectly clear), very rare occasion that I did actually bump into, or trip over someone else. Then, I would get angry with myself because I was then clearly a pillock who had, albeit briefly, come down to their level. Bad Danny; bad, bad (but not awful) Danny.

halls, festivals and such-like. They spoke words, so they'd learnt languages. Presumably they held jobs, had qualifications, people they cared for and who cared for them in return. They were not total pillocks.

Nor was it logical to conclude that they were complete pillocks just because they had the misfortune to get in my way. Even if it were utterly their responsibility, and they had not been looking where they were going, it would still not be logical to conclude they were complete pillocks, even if they did something we could both agree was stupid. Finally, this belief did not help me, it allowed me to demonise and judge other people. And it is so much easier to get angry with, and so much harder to empathise with other people when you're being judgemental.

Put-downs are not true, do not make sense and do not help you. Even if you utterly detest yourself (and, sadly, many people do), even if you feel like a complete waste of space, even if you feel that the achievements you do have do not mitigate this belief, you are still selling yourself a barrel-load of nonsensical, unhelpful lies.

These put-downs need to be replaced by something a whole lot more wholesome, kind, compassionate and accepting. Accepting of the self, of others and of life and all the things it contains.

It's almost time to look at your healthy beliefs.

The Four Thoughts That F*ck You Up: A Summary

So, there you have it, the four thoughts that disturb you are four unhealthy beliefs. There is a demand (using words such as 'must' and 'mustn't', 'should' and 'shouldn't' or 'got to' and 'have to'). Then there is a drama belief (also known as awfulising or catastrophising); and the 'I can't cope' belief (also known as low frustration tolerance). Finally, we have a put-down belief (also known as self-damning, other-damning or world-damning).

There is always a demand. If you are disturbed, says REBT, always look for the demand. Not everyone makes a drama, and if you are doing a drama in the face of one particular demand, don't automatically assume that you are doing one in the face of another different demand. Not everyone holds an I can't cope belief for every demand. Equally, not everybody holds a put-down belief, and if you are holding a put-down belief in the face of one demand, don't auto-matically assume that you are doing so again in the face of another demand.

Always look for the demand, always assume one is present if you are disturbing yourself. The other beliefs are assessed on a case-by-case basis.

Going back to timekeeping. Someone might be on a train believing 'I must be on time for everything and it is awful when I am not on time for everything'. Someone else could believe 'I must be on time for everything and I can't stand it when I am not on time for everything'. Some people will hold both a drama belief and an I can't cope belief in the face of 'I must be on time for everything'.

Someone else could be on the train believing 'I must be on time for everything and it's all my fault, I'm an idiot when I am not'. Someone else could be saying, 'I must be on time for everything, it's the bloody manager's fault when I am not.'

And someone else again could believe 'I must be on time for everything and it's the train company's fault when I am not, it is useless'.

And, someone else could be playing with the full deck, namely: 'I must be on time for everything, it is awful when I am not, I can't stand it when I am not and it's all my fault, I am an idiot when I am not'.

Thankfully, every single one of these unhealthy beliefs has a healthy and rational equivalent. You can have a desire or need, but the belief behind it can be rational. You can still rate the badness of things, but in a healthy way. You can still acknowledge frustration and the need to tolerate it, but in a helpful way. And you can still rate yourself, or others or world conditions, but in a much more kind and caring way.

It's time to meet the four thoughts that stop the unhealthy beliefs and that promote psychological wellbeing. They're the ones that will aid your mental health, that will help you think, feel and act in a much more rational way, that will stop you from fucking things up and, basically, prevent you from doing your head in.

How does that sound?

PART TWO

THE FOUR THOUGHTS THAT WILL FIX THEM

Flexible Preferences

The mental flexibility of the wise man permits him to keep an open mind and enables him to readjust himself whenever it becomes necessary for a change.

Malcolm X

Demands are rigid beliefs that disturb you. They are the rigid expression of a desire for something. When it comes to the four thoughts that fuck with your head, they sit at number one. Demands are not true, they do not make sense and they do not help you get the thing you demand you must have (in fact, they make it less likely that you will).

So, is there a way out of this madness? Can you fix that unhealthy thought? Can you correct the unhealthy demand and replace it with something more useful, helpful and rational? The answer is yes you can. Say hello to the flexible preference.

A 'preference' is a belief where you express what you would *like* to happen while, at the same time, accepting that it doesn't have to happen. You state your desire (I prefer XYZ) and then you negate the demand (but I don't have to have XYZ).

Your preference can take the form of 'I prefer', 'I wish', 'I hope' or 'I would like'; or words to that effect. But, you can't just say 'I prefer to have'. You have to negate your preference by adding 'but I don't have to have it'.

That bit is really important. If you just state your preference but do not negate it then, over time, you run the risk of turning it back into a demand. The 'but', and everything that comes after it, prevents that from happening.

And it is okay to hold a preference, because we all have preferences for things. Preferences for where we like to holiday, preferences for what food we like to eat, for how we like to be treated by others, for how we want life to treat us, where we want to be at any given time in life, what we want to achieve and so on, even preferences for how close we like people to be before we feel like they are invading our space.[1]

As long as we stick to our preferences, we remain psychologically healthy. Unfortunately, we human beings have a biological tendency to take our strongly held preferences and turn them into demands. The more important something is to us, the more likely we are to use words such as 'must' and 'mustn't' to express it.

This usually applies to the big stuff: respect, relationships, achievements (or lack thereof), life events and so on. In my practice, I used to say, 'Look, no one is going to disturb themselves over a cup of coffee.' But, then I had to stop saying that because someone did.

---

[1] And the distance attached to that preference can change depending on who it is applied to.

I had a client, a very exacting company CEO, who was very used to people executing his commands. When he said the proverbial 'jump', people literally jumped. When he said, 'Do it that way,' people did it exactly that way. He wasn't irrational exactly; he simply got away with being a demanding boss by being the boss. His rationality fell down, however, when it came to a simple cup of coffee. He liked a certain style, from a certain chain, with a certain type of non-dairy milk; all served a certain way with a certain attention to detail. If any of those elements failed to come in to play, he would lose his temper, shout, swear and kick chairs over. Not only was he angry in the moment, but he was also ashamed and embarrassed later on, and was spending a fortune on apology chocolates and flowers. 'I must have my coffee the way I want it,' he was saying, 'it's done my way at work and it must be done my way here.'

Except that in the coffee shop, he wasn't the CEO; he was the customer, and a very rude one at that.

This wasn't displaced anger (anger about something else, expressed somewhere else) and he wasn't stressed in other areas of his life (although we did explore this). He had simply extended his demandingness as a boss into an area in which he was not the boss.

In order to be able to show his face in his local coffee shop without hiding it behind a big bunch of carnations, he needed to accept that, as much as he liked his coffee a certain way, he did not *have* to have it a certain way.[2]

---

[2] Apparently carnations, roses, hyacinths, tulips, lily of the valley and orchids are flowers that say 'sorry'.

The preference is everything the demand is not. It's flexible and rational; it's way more realistic than the demand ever was, it makes much more sense to hold it and it will help you achieve your goal. Preferences are the route to psychological wellbeing. Embracing your preferences is how you fix your dogmatic demands.

It's perfectly fine to prefer to be in control, as long as you accept that you don't have to be in control, not all the time. It's perfectly fine to hope your partner treats you with respect, as long as you accept that they don't have to and probably won't treat you with respect all the time (especially if you are being as equally angry and disrespectful as they are). It's totally acceptable to want everything to be perfect, just so long as you accept that not everything is going to be tip-top, A+ and the best of the best. Not all the time.

You might be worried when control slips, or frustrated when your partner is not respecting you, or disappointed when your best efforts haven't quite reached the bar you set. But, these are much more rational expressions of emotion than, say, anxiety or anger or shame.

When you hold a preference, you will still react emotionally in the face of an adversity or a challenge but the emotion will be a healthy one. It will still be negative but it will be rational. This means that the thoughts, feelings and behaviours you exhibit will also be rational and, by that, we mean more in line with what you want or more helpful to you and to others.

For instance, someone who demands that their partner or friend must respect them will, most likely, be angry whenever they feel disrespected by that person. This means they are primed for any and all instances where respect is neither shown nor given. They may shout, or spoil for a fight, or demand, forcefully, to be respected. However, when you hold a preference for respect but also accept that your partner or friend doesn't have to respect you, you may be frustrated when respect is not forthcoming but not angry. You will feel different and you will behave differently. You will be a lot less loud and shouty for one thing, and much more calm and communicative.

And this is the curious thing: when you state what you prefer, but at the same time accept that you do not have to have the thing that you prefer, you make it much more likely that you will get it. Not guaranteed, but more likely.

Remember when I said that if you demand that you must pass your exam, you would probably make yourself anxious, revise badly, sleep poorly and not perform to the best of your ability come the day? Well, when you believe that you would prefer to pass the exam but also accept that you don't have to, then you will be more chilled about the same exam. Worried, yes, but not anxious. And so, your revision and sleep will be improved, which in turn will have a positive impact upon your performance on the day.

When you prefer respect, but accept that it does not have to be given, you think and feel and act in ways more likely to gain respect. When you prefer to be the best, but accept you don't have to be the best, you are still motivated to do well, but you are motivated while free from the fear and the stress of failure, which means you're more likely to do your best. As someone said in my clinic only the other day, 'I would still push myself, but I wouldn't push myself over the edge.' When you prefer (but don't demand) that life be better than it is, but also accept that it is what it is at the moment, you free your-self from depression. You also make it more likely that you will take steps to improve your lot.

The preference (plus the acknowledgement that you don't have to have the thing that you prefer) means you're more likely to receive positive emotional and behavioural results – not just for yourself, but also for others.

The first two parts of this book are inviting you to change the way you look at life and all of its problems. These chapters on healthy beliefs are asking you to adopt a different philoso-phy in the face of that life and its attendant problems.

As the famous nineteenth century essayist, philosopher, poet and transcendentalist, Ralph Waldo Emerson, once said: 'All life is an experiment.'[3] When you adopt the beliefs laid out here and in the following chapters, you may be surprised at the results. Some people feel a little daunted by this at first, and you may too, but you're quite safe. And, if you don't like the results, you are always free to return to your old ways of thinking.

But, have a go and notice. How do you feel when you drop your demands and adopt flexible preferences instead? How do you act? What do you do differently? Have you noticed a change in the way people respond to you?

And, more importantly, do you like those changes?

---

[3] Transcendentalists believe society and its institutions (especially political parties and organised religion) corrupt the purity of the individual. They claim that people are at their best when they are truly self-reliant and independent. For some strange reason, nei-ther politics nor religion like this philosophy very much.

An Important Thing about Preferences

Some people change their preferences in ways that sound rational, but aren't actually very rational at all. So, 'I prefer to be on time for everything, but I don't have to be' becomes 'I prefer to be on time for everything, but it's okay when I'm not'. Or it becomes 'I prefer to be on time for everything but it doesn't matter when I'm not.'

Some people do not have a thing for punctuality, they can't be on time to save their lives. Other people just don't care if they leave you waiting for an hour or so. They're the sort of people that can turn up really, really late and not even notice that you're fuming. 'Hey,' they say with a beguiling innocence, and then wonder why your face is all red and blotchy. (Someone with a preference for being on time is not one of those people.)

REBT will not try to change someone who cares about punctuality into someone who doesn't care about punctuality. That would be both weird and counter-productive. If you have a bit of a thing for being on time, it still won't be okay when you're not, even when you're holding a preference. It will still be important to you, because you prefer to be on time. However, it becomes not so important that you freak out about it.

By the same token, it will still matter to you if you are not on time. Again this is because you prefer to be on time. You won't like it, plus there could be negative consequences attached to your delay, but it won't be awful.

So, beware of 'it's okay' and 'it doesn't matter'. They have no place in your preferences. The only way to correctly express a preference is by also accepting that you don't have to have the thing that you prefer to get.

Some people worry that by adopting preferences, they are going to give up on pursuing their dreams, or get lazy and complacent, or become a bit of a pushover. None of these things are going to happen. If this is a concern of yours, then fear not and fret not as it is dealt with in the FAQ section of this book.

So, not only are preferences everything a demand is not, not only do they allow you to be who you are; but they also give you good psychological results.[4]

Back to Disputing

We challenge your unhealthy beliefs with those three rational questions:

'Is it true?'

'Does it make sense?'

'Does it help me?'

This clearly shows that they are not and do not. But, we also need to challenge your healthy beliefs in the same way. Why do you think that is? Why don't we just leave the healthy beliefs alone? Why do we challenge them as effectively, rationally and objectively as we do the unhealthy beliefs?

---

[4] And, by that, we mean you get more of what you want the way you want it, instead of more of what you don't want served in a way you also don't want.

Let's go back to my example of the scientist. So there I am, I have just successfully run an experiment that revolutionises our understanding of Einstein's theory of relativity and I'm thinking of myself as really rather clever.

So clever, in fact, that I want to get my experiment down on paper and published in a journal. So I take my results to my peers. The first thing they are going to ask for is the evidence. And, I have it. I present it. My work is meticulous and they are most impressed with the evidence I have shown. That's the first hurdle cleared. So the next attack is logical. Does my research make sense? Does my conclusion logically follow from my premise? If I can present logic, if I can demonstrate that my findings progress, logically, from one to the other, then publication is another step closer. Finally, we have the pragmatic question. Does my experiment help? Does it actually expand on what's gone before it and does it add anything new? Let's say it does, let's say it doesn't just go beyond what Einstein originally proposed, it totally blows it out of the water. Well, then, my peers are happy, I am happy, everybody is happy and into a journal my research paper goes. Free Champagne for everybody!

These disputing questions are excellent for challenging things, not only to see what falls apart, but to also see what holds up against such intensive scrutiny. After all, we don't want you to replace one weak and shoddy fall-apart belief with another, equally weak and shoddy fall-apart belief now, do we? So, let's apply that way of thinking to a preference.

Take the healthy belief of, 'I prefer to be on time, but I don't have to be on time'. Here you have stated your preference and, at the same time, you have negated your demand. It is realistic in that, while it takes into account that you are someone with 'a bit of a thing' for punctuality, it also acknowledges that delays can and will occur. It's true that you prefer punctuality, but it's also true that you will be late sometimes. It's much more logical to accept that, as much as you like to be on time, there are always occasions where you won't be. The conclusion 'but I don't have to be on time for everything' logically flows from your premise, 'I prefer to be on time'. Taken separately, they are both rational statements; and one connects to the other. Here, your reason is sound.

This belief is sensible, and it would help you deal with the inevitable delays you will face to your journey times in a much more calm and productive manner. You won't like the delay because you prefer to be on time (and you don't have to like it), but you can deal with it in a rational fashion.

As I write this, I am on another train journey similar to the one I mentioned earlier, only this time I am on the return: from London Paddington to Bristol Temple Meads. And, guess what? I'm delayed again. The preference is definitely helping me right now, in that while I am a little vexed, I am also calm enough to be writing this as I deal with said delay. I wish I could say the same of some of the people around me.

Now, take the healthy version of my anger problem that I brought up in the classroom all those years ago: 'I would prefer it if other people didn't get in my way, but there is no reason why other people must not get in my way'.

This acknowledges who I am. I am most definitely the sort of person who prefers other people not to barge into him, not to bump into him and not to trip him up. As I said earlier, if I had my way, all shops and train stations would mysteriously empty upon my entrance, allowing me to shop and commute with freedom and ease. I'd be like one of those celebrities that orders an entire shop floor emptied just so they could buy a top, or go to the loo, in private. Sadly, I live in the real world, and that's full of people, everywhere, all of them getting in each other's way. All the people who have ever bumped into me are evidence that that is so.

'I would prefer it if other people didn't get in my way, but there is no reason why other people must not get in my way' is way more logical than 'I would prefer it if other people didn't get in my way, so they must not'. My preference is rational, and my acceptance that I don't have to get the thing that I prefer is equally rational, therefore one can be concluded from the other.

And, if I truly believed my preference, it would help me. It did help me. It has helped me. It helps me still, today. I am mildly frustrated, or annoyed, or vexed even, when people do actually get in my way or bump into me, but I am rarely ever angry. I am in control of my emotions; my emotions are not in control of me. Plus, I have lost that nagging little worry that one day someone, somewhere, was either going to thump me or have me arrested.[5]

The most I ever get, and I have to really be bumped into quite a lot in a short space of time to get there, is mildly sarcastic. 'Thank you for doing that,' I say. 'Thank you for getting in my way.' Although, mostly, I say, 'That's quite alright,'

---

[5] No one wants to say, 'Yes, Your Honour,' when asked if they have ever growled at someone like a bear.

whenever someone says 'sorry' for bumping into me. I even say it when they don't.

We are our preferences. They are our truths. They help us define ourselves and relate ourselves to other people.

We communicate our preferences on a daily basis. When we say we like something, it's pretty safe to assume it's true. Evidence doesn't just have to be factual; it can also be experiential. If I walk into a travel shop and talk to the agent about Mauritius and the Maldives, but the agent shows me Margate and Bognor Regis, they've clearly invalidated my exotic holiday preferences, I am liable to walk out in a huff and they're hardly likely to be enjoying any commission from a holiday booked via me.

Let's say you invite me round for dinner, and you call me up a couple of days beforehand to ascertain my culinary likes and dislikes. You ask me, 'What do you prefer, lamb or beef?' And I pick beef. I tell you I love steak. Hopefully, you're going to serve me steak. Then you ask me, 'What do you prefer, sticky toffee pudding or tiramisu?' And I reply, 'Oh my god, I love sticky toffee pudding.' Then, hopefully, that's exactly what you'll serve me. You don't challenge my preferences; you accept them as my reality.[6]

The preference certainly helped my carnation-buying CEO client. As far as I know, he never needed to buy a coffee-related apology bouquet ever again.

---

[6] Sadly, this understanding does not apply to children. 'Eat your broccoli,' you say. 'But, I don't like broccoli,' they say. 'Yes you do,' you say, 'now eat it all up or you won't get your sticky toffee pudding.'

So, there you have it, unhealthy demands mess you up . . . they trigger anger, anxiety, depression and a whole host of other unhealthy negative emotions and unhelpful behaviours while flexible preferences will help promote a much healthier and happier you. They also work amazingly well on other people too. On your mothers and fathers, on partners and on your sons and daughters.

It's amazing how much nicer and more cooperative people are when, instead of telling them they have to do it like this or that they must do it like that, you simply offer it up as a preference. More than one client over the years has turned their rebellious young son or daughter into a dream, just by saying, 'Look, you don't have to do this, but Mummy/Daddy/primary caregiver would prefer it if you did.'

Not all the time though as, sometimes, you will still have to scream, 'Just bloody do it, because I'm your bloody Mum/Dad/primary caregiver.' Only, now you can do it safe in the knowledge that you just issued a conditional demand: ABC must happen (do what I say) or else XYZ will happen (you will be in serious trouble, young man/woman/person).

And, the great thing about preferences is that when people hold them, they are more rational in the expression of those other beliefs too. When people hold to their preferences, they are also more able to keep a sense of perspective in times of trouble, which brings us on to our next healthy belief . . .

Possessing Perspective

> I am not afraid of the storms, for I am learning to sail my ship.
>
> Louisa May Alcott

Would you like to see things as they truly are, without blowing them out of proportion or making them worse than they actually are? No matter how dire the consequences, or how horrible the situation you find yourself in, would you like to keep a sense of objectivity in times of adversity? You would? Great, then welcome to the world of 'perspective', also known in REBT as 'anti-awfulising'.

Okay, so the term sounds a bit *Star Trek*. Well, it does to me at least.[1] 'We've lost containment in the anti-awfulising chamber, Captain. Everything's gone critical. If I give her any more, she'll blow!'

---

[1] So too does 'Nutrileum', but, not so long ago, that was just a made-up name for a particular constituent of a certain shampoo brand. Although, a spokesperson for said brand called it 'an innovative association of a cationic silicone derivative and camelina oil'.

And words to that effect – except that here, nothing can get critical, and nothing will get to the point where it blows. With anti-awfulising, things would never escalate that far. Anti-awfulising is a healthy, rational rating of the badness of any given situation or of your demand not being met, or of that rigid, absolute law in your head being broken.

What we are acknowledging is that we live in a world where bad things do indeed happen and, when they do, you most certainly don't have to like them. The world does indeed contain things that you don't like and, sometimes, you do just have to suck it up. And that's not nice. But, neither is it the end of the world. Nothing is ever the end of the world, except for the end of the world.

If you fail to get your promotion, if someone is not respecting you, if crowds of people get in your way, if your train is not on time, it will not be a good thing. (Especially if you wanted the promotion, like it when people respect you, don't like crowds of people getting in your way and are keen on punctuality). These are bad things. But, you can think of worse: no one is ill and no one has died; you still have food on your plate and a roof over your head.

So here, bad just means bad, no more and no less.

The English language is replete with idioms that encapsulate this particular belief system: 'worse things happen at sea', 'the best-laid plans of mice and men often go astray', 'the darkest hour is just before the dawn' or 'that's the way the cookie crumbles'. Even *'c'est la vie,'* (which the English probably use far more than the French), or simply 'shit happens'. All are, in essence, just ways of understanding that things are never as bad as they seem.

Anti-awfulising states, very calmly, that while it may be bad when you don't get what you want, it is never the worst thing that you can think of, or the worst thing that could actually happen. We all walk around with a scale of badness in our heads, comprised mainly of bad things that have actually happened, but also of things that could happen. My scale of badness would look very different to yours, and your scale of badness would look very different to your best mate's scale, and so on. And that scale is an ever-evolving thing. The items it contains go up and down that scale in relation to all the other bad things that occur, or could occur, in your life.

For instance, some people are not that bothered about failing an exam, so that would sit very low down on their personal scale of badness, while other people would think failing an exam (as it is important to them) a very bad thing indeed. And you have every right to rate things as bad as you want to rate them. However, whatever you put on that scale, and wherever you put it, you can always think of something worse. To do so allows you to keep a sense of perspective in all things and in all situations.

When you hold an anti-awfulising belief, when you have that sense of perspective, something is always the molehill and never the mountain; it doesn't matter what the crisis is, you have not given it any added drama.

People who awfulise or dramatise, who blow things out of proportion, are prone to run around like headless chickens whenever problems occur, or panic, worrying about all the other horrible things that could happen because of the thing they have just rated as awful. People who can see things as bad but not awful, more often than not either don't worry about it because it's not that big a deal, or don't worry about it because it hasn't happened yet, or they remain solution-focussed if something has happened and needs sorting out. Life becomes remarkably free from drama when you look at things that way.

And, doesn't that just sound, well, nice? After all, who wouldn't want a drama-free life? But, how do you get one? How do you get yourself there? How do you stop yourself going critical whenever there is a crisis?

Don't Forget Disputing

Perhaps, unsurprisingly, it's back to those three, rational, disputing questions. Believing something to be bad, but not awful, is not only provable with evidence, it is also demonstrably logically and decidedly more helpful than its unhealthy alternative (especially if your goal is to remain calm in times of challenge, or to keep your cool when all around you are losing theirs).

Remember my bald men? Well, 'being bald is awful' has now become 'being bald is bad, but it is not awful'.

This belief is true. If you are the sort of person that wishes they had more hair on their head than they do, then you are not going to like it when you don't have more hair on your head than you do. So, for you, it is a bad thing. There could also be negative consequences to your lack of hair. The evidence those guys gave in the therapy room – the proof I mentioned earlier, such as not liking it, feeling less of a man, not getting the partner they wanted, being judged, blocking the sink with moulting hair, and so on – is evidence that it is bad being bald.

They did not like it (and they do not have to like it either). If someone you like does not like bald men, and then rejects you because of it, that is not a good thing.

It is a bad thing, so 'being bald' will exist on your scale of badness. But, you can think of worse things. You can think of so many things that are 'more bad' than you being bald, each one more or less bad than the other things, depending where they sit on your personal spectrum of badness. You can also offer up good things (Jason Statham! Bruce Willis! Salon savings!). Awful does not exist.[2]

It also makes sense. Saying it's bad being bald is rational (especially if you are the sort of person that likes hair on their head). However, saying it isn't awful is also rational (even though you are the sort of person that likes hair on their head). One notion (but it is not awful) logically follows from the other (being bald is bad).

As a belief, 'being bald is bad but it is not awful' will help you. You are no longer blowing things out of proportion, for a start; you are seeing things as they are. You will have gained a sense of perspective. These are the people who stop spending a fortune on hair loss treatments and invest in a pair of hair clippers instead. They learn to live with a No. 1 or No. 2, and wear hats when it's cold and sun cream when it's hot.

These are the people who calmly realise that while some people find coiffure sexy and some people find bald sexy, almost everyone finds happiness and confidence sexy. And

---

[2] Although, more than one person has pointed out that what they save in hair cuts they spend in back wax treatments because, whilst genetics can taketh away in some areas, it can also giveth in others.

so, they work on that instead. Anti-awfulising is awesome at helping you zero in on a solution to any problem.

For every person in that company I once worked in that screamed 'nightmare' whenever something went wrong, there was another person that calmly looked at the problem, then fixed the problem and then got everything back on track. I was one of them. But, we all have our Achilles' heel. And, by now, you are well-acquainted with one of mine so, back to my belief about crowds, but this time rationalised: 'It's bad when people get in my way, but it is not awful.'

This belief is true. It's definitely true for me. Even today; with many years of REBT under my belt, I still don't like crowds and I still don't like it when people get in my way; my frustration in crowded places proves that this is so. And, just as importantly, I don't have to like them, I don't have to strive to be the sort of person that will ever like them. However, as I can think of so many things that are worse (including things that have actually happened to me), it's also true that it isn't awful when they do get in my way. Saying it's bad, understanding that I don't like crowds and never will, is rational, and concluding that it isn't awful is equally rational, therefore this belief makes sense: one point (other people getting in my way is not awful) logically follows from the other point (I don't like other people getting in my way). It also helps me. More specifically, it helps me keep my anger under control, it allows me to see the problem as it is and it allows me to go into crowded places, if I want to or need to, without kicking off.[3]

---

[3] To the relief of many.

It still doesn't make me a good shopping companion though. As shopping also sits on my personal scale of badness (i.e., the things I don't like to do and don't have to like doing).

A Word or Two about Trauma

When something traumatic happens, you are allowed to be dysfunctional. You are allowed to be angry and depressed and anxious and numb and all of it. REBT is not necessarily the right thing for people who have just experienced trauma.

As mentioned earlier, if you are going through a current or very recent traumatic event, counselling would be a better place for you to start. Being held in a safe space while processing your emotions would be more appropriate. Although being rational can help, it also helps to scream and yell and rail against the world as you process the traumatic event.[4] Although the healthy, rational beliefs outlined in this book can and will help you to be more resilient emotionally and physically in the face of trauma, you are allowed to be all 'must' and 'mustn't' and 'awful' and 'nightmare' about it in the immediacy of it.

REBT is for after, for later on down the line, if you haven't processed the traumatic event or haven't moved on from it. It's for if you are stuck, months or even years after the fact, still angry or depressed, or anxious or guilty.

If you tell a person who's just lost someone they love that it's not the end of the world, and that they'll soon

---

[4] However, there is a specific form of CBT known as Trauma-focussed CBT that's proven to be very effective indeed.

meet someone else, you'll probably get a wallop.[5] That said, I work with the employees of several train operating companies and, among the many stresses and strains particular to this line of work, they have the stress of suicide. More specifically, when someone has used a train as their particular method for ending it. This is a very stressful and traumatic event, not only for the family of the person concerned, but also for the passengers on the train, the staff managing the train, the people who have to come and sort everything out and, in particular, very stressful for the train driver involved.

However, for every train driver who takes plenty of time off work to heal and recover, or who comes to therapy to help them expedite that process, there is a train driver who takes it in his stride and who is ready to return to work before they've even been declared fit for duty. They're not inhuman and they don't lack empathy, they've just managed to look at what has happened in a way that hasn't disturbed them.

It's part of the job, they say; they hope it doesn't happen to them, but they accept that it can and probably will and that, as bad as it is, it is not the worst thing they can think of. Some people can and do experience relief by being rational in the immediacy of a traumatic event.

That's enough about trauma for now, so back to those beliefs.

To work out if you are awfulising a demand, ask yourself, 'When I am at my most disturbed, am I awfulising? Am I

---

[5] You'll definitely be off their Christmas card list.

making it worse than it is?' Imagining yourself when at your most disturbed is important. If you don't, you will be tempted to give the rational answer (no, I'm not). We want the answer that the really angry; the really depressed; the really panic-stricken you will give. Because, although we can all be rational, rationality leaves the room when we hold a demand. It checks out, it goes on a long holiday.[6]

Also, check your feelings. Check what they are telling you. If something feels awful, terrible or catastrophic, then behind that feeling is the belief that it is awful, terrible or catastrophic.

Similarly, if you identify an awfulising belief, you can automatically assume there is a demand. So, for instance, if you say, 'The way my boss speaks to me is just awful,' and you're pretty disturbed about it, you can automatically assume that you hold the demand 'my boss must not speak to me like that'.

When you have identified a demand, you can turn it into a preference. When you have identified an awfulising belief, you can automatically assume the demand is present, and formulate a preference and an anti-awfulising belief, such as: 'I would prefer that my boss did not speak to me like that, but there is no reason why they mustn't; it's bad when they do talk to me like that, but it is not awful'.

Scales of Badness: a Caveat

When you think of that bad thing that happened to you placed on a scale of badness, relative to all the other things that are

---

[6] And it doesn't send a text.

less bad than it and more bad than it, please do not disturb yourself further by worrying about all the other bad things that could happen, but haven't happened yet and are hardly likely to happen anyway.[7]

Let's say, for instance, that you find a strange lump on your body. An awfuliser will immediately jump to all the worst case scenarios: it's cancer, it's malignant, it's inoperable and it's terminal. They will probably Google symptoms that confirm their diagnosis and then make themselves even more anxious than they already were. They will make a doctor's appointment and be anxious in the lead-up to it. They won't be satisfied with the doctor's opinion and won't rest until they've had a biopsy and a diagnosis. The words 'malignant' and 'terminal' will still be at the forefront of their minds. More importantly, they will act as if these things have already happened. They will add these things to the list of things they are getting disturbed about.

An anti-awfuliser, however, looks at the same strange lump in a completely different way. They will be more likely to stick to a neutral diagnosis, such as 'I have a lump'. They won't go Googling symptoms, but they will monitor the situation and possibly make a doctor's appointment. A little concern may be in order, but that's about it. They will then patiently wait for the doctor's diagnosis and also agree and accept what they are told. If the word 'biopsy' is mentioned they may again feel concerned, but they won't be anxious as there is nothing, as yet, to worry about. A biopsy, you see, is not a diagnosis.

---

[7] Anxiety keeps you worrying about a great many things, most of which will never happen.

I happen to know this personally. Many years ago, a strange blue lump appeared on my lower lip, ever-so-slightly on the inside, and it did not go away. I didn't worry, but I did eventually go to the doctor. 'Ooh,' said the doctor, 'I had better send you to a specialist.' I duly went. 'Ooh,' said the specialist, 'we had better take a biopsy.' A biopsy was taken. I still did not worry. 'Ooh,' said the specialist, when the results came back, 'we had better get that removed.' My worry increased a little at this point, but I still didn't get anxious.

Two days before the surgery, I was invited to meet the surgeon. 'Are you sure you want to have this procedure?' he asked, which confused me. Surely it was a dangerous lump and needed *poste haste* removal? The answer was no. It turned out that what I had was nothing more than a benign fatty lump. Removing it was problematic in that surgery on the lip, being the warm, moist and sensitive area that it is, is both painful and prone to frequent reinfection, plus the lump would probably come back again. Equally, it would probably just disappear of its own volition.

Given that, I elected to leave well alone and one day I woke up and realised that it had gone, but I had paid it such little attention that I couldn't exactly say when it had gone. Anti-awfulising had dictated that, while a little caution was necessary, anxiety was not. In hindsight, though, I think I would have questioned the specialist and the biopsy results a little more thoroughly than I had. Concern is one thing, but laissez-faire is another.

One of my friends always says, 'Worse things happen at sea,' whenever something bad happens. And he means it. He is pretty unflappable. This is anti-awfulising in action.

I have another friend, one who used to lurch from one calamity to another, getting very depressed and very anxious in equal measure (either on rotation or altogether). I never went through any formal therapy with her as it's not ethical to therapise people you know. However, I did drip-feed her REBT on a regular basis: over the phone, over lunch, over a pint or two down the pub, and so on. I challenged her every 'awful' and 'nightmare' and helped her to see a healthier alternative. Over the course of a few short months, her side of the conversation went something like: 'Is that REBT? That's REBT, is it? I don't think much of that. It sounds stupid. I know what you're doing. It won't work on me. It's not working you know,' and so on. Until one fine day, when she swept into the bar we had arranged to meet up in, sat down and, before we'd even exchanged hellos, said, 'I hate you.'

I smiled angelically and asked, 'Why's that?' with a wide-eyed innocence.

She had gone to have a meltdown at work over some situation or other but, just as her emotions were about to escalate, she'd recalled one of our conversations. She heard my voice say, 'Is it really that terrible; can you not think of anything worse? How does that actually stack up against the other bad things that have happened to you?' And that was it. That was enough. Her dramatic reaction was deflated.

I have a further friend still who, despite my best efforts, remains one of life's awfulisers. Regardless of all the drip-feeding, he still takes things to the extreme. This case highlights something that is as true of life as it is of therapy: sadly, you just can't help everyone.

Over the years, people have argued that the end of the world would be an awful thing and argue therefore that this rational sense of perspective has a ceiling. They have tried to present Armageddon in all its forms as a disputing fail, or as some kind of dramatic *fait accompli*.

However, with a sense of perspective, you can open up a whole conversation on all the different ways that the world could end, and which ending would be more bad that another. With a sense of perspective, you can also evidence some good that will come out of the end of the world. If it's the end of the world as we know it (due, say, to climate change and the collapse of our ecosystem), then the Earth will lie fallow for a few millennia (as it's done several times before) and then start anew. However, if it's the world exploding to bits due to a massive calamity then that's more bad, but it is not beyond the realms of possibility that chemical fragments from our world will travel across the vastness of space and, eventually, seed new life on a world far from here.[8] So, even the end of the world isn't awful, it's just bad, to varying degrees.

So, there you have it. Anti-awfulising, the rational rating of the badness of any given situation (or of the badness of your demands not being met or being broken), where something is bad but not awful, is true. It does make sense and it does help you: it helps you to remain calm and steadfast in the face of any given difficulty. With it, you gain a sense of perspective,

---

[8] This is known as 'panspermia' and it's theorised that life on Earth originated from microorganisms and chemical constituents that travelled here from space. Possibly from another world, and one that was possibly blown-up due to indigenous incompetence.

and you see things as they truly are, without blowing them out of proportion.

When you think of things that way, when it's the molehill and never the mountain, the crisis without the drama, you see things as they are, on that scale of badness, but in relation to all the other bad things that have happened, are happening or could ever happen in your life.

Awfulising leaves you quagmired, with nowhere else left to go, while anti-awfulising allows you to see beyond, through the bad thing and out the other side to either acceptance of the situation as it currently stands, or to its eventual solution.

If you get really good at anti-awfulising, you'll be able to take any and all challenging, negative events in your stride, just like my unflappable, 'worse things happen at sea' friend. Holding this belief, then, will forever give you a sense of perspective.

But, let's build on that, shall we? As with Doing a Drama, so too with an attack of the I Can't Copes. There is a healthy alternative, a way of looking at testing times, stressful situations and challenging circumstances that allow you to carry on, despite the adversity, all without dying, throwing a strop, falling apart or disappearing in a huge puff of exasperation . . .

The I Can Copes

Life begins at the end of your comfort zone.

Neale Donald Walsch

Instead of low frustration tolerance we have (perhaps unsurprisingly) high frustration tolerance (HFT), also known as 'it may be difficult if I don't get what I want, but I know I can cope with not getting what I want', AKA 'it is difficult to deal with, but I can stand it' and sometimes, simply, 'resilience'.

Resilience became a buzzword in stress management circles a while back, and also in business management workshops. Not so long ago, people liked seminars and keynote speeches with titles such as 'Building Emotional and Mental Resilience' and 'How Your Workforce Remains Resilient During the Third Quarter,' but that star is fading a little which is a shame. Because whenever and wherever anyone talks about resilience, or emotional or mental toughness, they are talking about high frustration tolerance. And it's an important thing to develop, not only in a person, but also in your psyche and your personnel.

We have idioms in the English language that encapsulate the notion of I Can Cope: 'whatever doesn't kill you makes you stronger' and 'when the going gets tough, the tough get going.'[1] We also have karaoke classics that highlight this principle – people are fond of belting out 'Stronger (What Doesn't Kill You)' by Kelly Clarkson as well as that certain HFT eponymous track by Billy Ocean. But, how do they do that? When the going gets tough, why do some people get going, while others fall apart?

Looking at it through the filter of REBT, people that fall apart believe that they *can't* cope when the going gets tough, while the people that don't fall apart believe they *can* cope when the going gets tough. The important thing to acknowledge here is that the going still got tough. It didn't get any easier, just because you're one of the tough. Because things do get difficult, life presents you with challenges and you are often taken out of your comfort zone, and these things are not always pleasant things. With high frustration tolerance, we do not deny that the going has indeed got more than a little tough, we simply acknowledge that you can deal with it, we point out that you have dealt with tough things before in the past and we use that to predict that you will deal with tough things again in the future.

When your goals are thwarted, it will be frustrating. Difficult people are difficult to deal with. Failing at something you wanted to succeed in will be challenging. Saying no to something you have a bit of a predilection for (be it a fine bottle of Merlot or everything there is on the dessert menu) will be very uncomfortable, but saying 'no' will not kill you.

---

[1] My personal favourite is 'Whatever doesn't kill you gives you a sick sense of humour and some seriously weird coping strategies'. Some of those coping strategies you may want to work on with REBT; others you may simply accept as part of who you are and some you may even appreciate despite the weirdness.

If it doesn't kill you, it is something you can cope with. It may not feel like it, but you can. It might be difficult, it might be challenging, it might be extreme but, if it hasn't killed you, then you can cope. As I said earlier in this book, you have survived every single challenging event in your life so far. Even when you said you couldn't stand it, you were standing it.

I had a client, a project manager with a team of five. Only, he couldn't trust his team to do things to his standards so he was forever taking the elements of the project for which they were responsible off them and doing the work himself. Which meant that A: he was always working late while his team went home on time; B: he was literally doing the work of six people; and, also C: he was very tired, very stressed and more than a little bit resentful of his team and their lack of support. When I asked him why he just didn't put the work back on his team and let them get on with it he said, 'Oh no, I couldn't cope with that.' So, we worked on his high frustration tolerance. His belief was: 'I would like to do it myself, but I don't have to do it myself, I will find handing the work back difficult, but I know I can stand it'. And we got him to hand the project elements back to those responsible for them, and then tolerate both the frustration of trusting his team and the frustration of them not getting it quite how he wanted it to be.

As he did this, a surprising thing happened. Well, surprising to him but not to me. The productivity of his team increased, as did the quality of their work.

He had unwittingly taught his team that, no matter what they did or did not do, he would take their efforts off their hands and complete it for them. So they had learnt to do a half-assed job, safe and sure in the knowledge that they would not have to repeat the task. Once he started handing the work back and asking them to work late to get it done to spec, the attitude of his team changed completely. Few people like working late, especially when it's to do what they've already done. More importantly, my client learnt to trust his team, delegate more, go home on time and improve the quality of his life.

Believing something to be difficult, but bearable, is true. Whether it is a person, a deadline or a demanding job. Your stress, your anxiety, your depression or your unhealthy coping strategies are proof that it is difficult, but the fact that you are alive to not deal with it as well as you would like to be dealing with it is proof positive that you can stand it. Saying that you find something difficult, challenging, frustrating or pressurising is rational, and saying that you can deal with, cope with and bear this challenge or difficulty is equally rational. Therefore, one logically flows from the other. Finally, believing that something is difficult but bearable, believing that you can cope with challenge and adversity will help you. It empowers you. It emboldens you, and it keeps you on course. In short, just getting on with it, in whatever way works best, becomes your coping strategy. You become your coping strategy because you become resilient to what Shakespeare called the 'slings and arrows of outrageous fortune'. You will have all the emotional and mental toughness that you need.

Take my now healthy belief about crowds: 'I find it difficult to deal with when other people get in my way but, I know I can stand it'. This belief is true. It is true that I find it difficult. Some people don't. They don't mind crowds, they don't mind getting bumped into at all.[2]

---

[2] The weirdos.

But, that's not me. To this day, I still find crowded places a little vexing. Even though I no longer mutter, shout at, growl like a bear, or shove people out of the way, I'm not all perfect calm and poise. When people do bump into me or trip me up, I find it frustrating. This is who I am. This is my truth. It is equally true that I can stand the difficulty of being bumped into. It has not killed me. I do not disappear in a flash of exasperation. Saying I find it difficult is rational, saying that I can cope with the difficulty is equally rational. One statement then logically flows from the other. And it has most definitely helped me over the years to believe this. I can venture out into crowded places if I want to or need to, I can cope with a visit to the shopping mall. If I avoid rush hour, it is simply because I can and because it is a sensible thing to do but I also know that if you place me in a rush-hour scenario, I won't get angry about it. I can cope. I'm happy, my friends are happy and the people that bump into me are happy too. 'I'm sorry,' they say. 'It's okay,' I reply.

Also, knowing that you can cope with something doesn't mean that you have to cope with it if you don't want to. This is a good thing. More than one person has come to see me, signed off sick from work with stress, only to return to work with a full conviction in their healthy beliefs and realise that, while they could indeed cope with the pressures of the job they were currently doing, they didn't have to. And, more importantly, they didn't want to. They then made the very rational decision to look for another, far less stressful, form of employment.

There is a whole world of difference between not doing something because you don't believe you can cope with it, and not doing something simply because you don't want to cope with it. I have proved I can cope with people getting in my way, but I will still avoid them if I can. With this new modus operandi of not being angry when people got in my way was set, I was free. Free to choose. Free to go into the crowded place if I wanted to or needed to, but also equally free not to. Especially if I had neither want nor need.

But what about things that are unavoidable or the things you have no choice over?

Well, it's back to the bald men on this one. Many of them did believe that being bald was unbearable, and so we had a lot of work to do on their healthy, high frustration tolerance alternative: 'I find being bald difficult to deal with, but I know I can stand it'. This belief was true for them. They did find it difficult. Their depressive episodes, their anxieties, insecurities and other issues proved that, as did the comb-overs and the mourning over the loss of an ever-changing, à la mode hairstyle. But, it was also true that they were alive and, usually, in my office bemoaning their lack of hair. No one has ever died of being bald.[3]

Saying that they found it difficult to deal with was rational, saying that they could stand the difficulty of being bald was equally rational. One belief logically flowed from the other belief. Given that male pattern baldness (which is the most common type of hair loss) usually starts in the late twenties and early thirties and affects around half of all men by the age of 50, it makes complete sense to believe this. Otherwise the male population would be decimated on a regular basis.

---

[3] Apart from a bizarre spate of deaths in Mozambique in 2017, where bald men were being killed because of the belief that their heads contained gold. No, really, they were. But here, their baldness did not kill them, other people killed them for being bald.

And boy did it help. It helped lift them out of their depressions, it helped them control their anxieties, to get their confidence back, to feel more secure, to believe in themselves, to go out and find partners if they were single, or stop worrying that their partners would leave them if they weren't and, often, to stop spending hundreds, if not thousands, of pounds on hair loss drugs and more besides.

The only things in this world that you can't stand are the things that kill you. If it doesn't kill you then you can cope with it, no matter how difficult it is. Being bald won't kill you, but someone clubbing you over the head to get at the gold stored inside it will do the trick.

And, no matter what it is, nor how difficult it is, it won't last forever. There's another expression that encapsulates the I Can Copes. 'This too shall pass' is not only a wise and venerable reflection on the ephemeral nature of the human condition, but also another strong reminder that you have so far survived 100 per cent of the stuff life has thrown at you.

Admittedly, being bald lasts a lifetime, but being depressed about being bald does not have to. Japanese writer Haruki Murakami once famously said, 'Pain is inevitable, suffering is optional.' When you believe you can't stand something, you will suffer the inevitable, but, when you believe something is difficult but bearable, you will weather the inevitable with either a little bit of suffering, or none at all. And, more importantly, you will weather it with fortitude.

This notion of I Can Cope also applies to those kissing cousins mentioned in the chapter on low frustration tolerance. Here, 'I can't be bothered' becomes 'I will find this thing tedious, or boring, but I know I can be bothered'. While 'I can't believe it' becomes 'while I find this information difficult to process, I can believe it'. Again, these beliefs are true, make sense and will help you.

Things can be boring and tedious. For every student that loves getting to grips with a thesis, there are a dozen who'd rather be down the pub. For every project manager who can't leave a project alone, there are more than a few who'd rather be at home watching the television. Housework is dull; cleaning the car and the fish tank equally dull. Life is full of tedium, but tedium doesn't kill you. No one has ever died of boredom, despite what people claim. And, if you have done a boring thing once before, you can do a boring thing once again and again and again; therefore, it is equally true that you can be bothered. Saying something is boring (if you do indeed find it boring) is rational. Saying you can be bothered to do the boring thing is equally rational, so one statement logically flows from the other. And this belief would help you. It would help you to get started in time, it would help you to tackle things one step at a time. It would help you start a task or project on time and finish on time without waiting for the stress of the looming deadline as your prime motivator to start.

By the by, if you Google 'has anyone died of . . .', then boredom comes out as the top suggestion. And science has some definite things to say on the subject. People do not die of boredom, but they do die of the unhealthy lifestyles that boredom can facilitate.

Which brings us back to the 'but' flipping.

What will happen if you say, 'I am bored, but I can be bothered to go to the gym.' Or, 'I find cooking tedious, but I can be bothered to cook using fresh ingredients?' Hello, healthy lifestyle is what will happen.

It's the same with 'I can't believe it' – something may be difficult to comprehend, but you can believe it. And, if something happened, it is true. You have the fact of its occurrence but, experientially, you have evidence of finding it hard to get your head around. Saying you find something difficult to get your head around is rational, but believing you can believe it is also rational, so one logically follows from the other. And it will definitely help you. You'll be able to get your head around the thing that happened faster, for a start and, if it's something you need to recover from (either physically or mentally), you'll begin that process of recovery a whole lot sooner.

When you believe that something is difficult, but that you can cope with it; when you believe you can deal with the boring thing; when you acknowledge the shocking event and comprehend it, life becomes easier. And it does so because you become stronger and more resilient.

Remember, low frustration tolerance strips away your healthy coping strategies and allows unhealthy coping strategies to creep in (such as avoidance, alcohol, drugs and so on). When you hold a high frustration tolerance belief, you are your own healthy coping strategy. Maybe you'll let it go, because it wasn't worth getting stressed about in the first place. Maybe you'll go home on time more often because it's just work and it will still be there in the morning. Maybe you'll go to the gym instead of the pub, maybe you'll go out with friends instead of sitting at home all alone in the dark, feeling drained. Maybe you'll trim your hair right down and be blatantly, unmistakably bald. Who knows? But, whatever decision you make on how you will deal with it, it will be the right one for you.

I can't help but wonder what university counselling departments would be like if their students arrived already believing that A: nothing was the end of the world, and B: they can cope with whatever student life throws at them. Similarly, I wonder if we'd still be the number one country in the developing world for work stress if the entire workforce believed the same things.

I do know that REBT has helped plenty of students deal with both school and university. It has also helped plenty of people go back to the same jobs they were signed off work sick from.

But it doesn't mean you have to stick with situations and people you don't want to. That would not be healthy or therapeutic. This is because, sometimes, not doing that thing you don't want to do is a healthy coping strategy, while not doing that thing because you believe you can't cope is always an unhealthy coping strategy.

As I mentioned earlier, I've indirectly helped people find new jobs because they've gone back to work and realised that while they can cope with what work is throwing at them, no sane person would want to and so they've moved on to something less demanding of their time.[4]

Once my 'Just get it fucking done, will you?' lady had shifted from 'I can't cope when people don't do it the way I want it to be done' to 'I will find it difficult to deal with when

---

[4] Much to the surprise of their employer, especially when they had paid for the therapy in the first place; which only goes to show that The Law of Unintended Consequences (that actions of people always have effects that are unanticipated or unintended) is actually a thing.

people don't do it the way I want it to be done, but I know I can stand it', both her work life and her home life become a whole lot more pleasurable and relaxed, not only for her, but also for her co-workers and family. There was significantly less swearing for a start.

That said, later on in this book you are going to discover that swearing, when used correctly that is, can be both a great stress reliever and a wonderful aid to thinking rationally.

Earlier, I discussed the four types of I Can't Cope – emotional intolerance (where you can't deal with emotional distress), entitlement intolerance (where you can't stand unfairness or frustrated gratification), discomfort intolerance (where you can't deal with difficulties or hassles) and, finally, achievement intolerance (where you can't deal with not achieving your goals).

Put those through the filter of 'it's difficult to deal with but I know I can cope' and what do you come up with? You will be better able to cope with the demands of your job, with difficult-to-deal-with people, with not achieving your goals and with situations not going your way. Essentially, there won't be much that life can throw at you that you won't be able to take in your stride.

We are meant to be emotional human beings, but some people believe they can't handle their emotions, while others haven't been taught how to handle them. Some even turn to suicide and self-harm as a way to deal with their more troubling emotions. I've found that, often, when people are taught that they can cope with their difficult emotions, they naturally develop healthier ways of coping. People who can cope with difficult people become excellent at either mediating, or letting it go over their heads, or both. Sports people are the epitome of 'I can cope with being thwarted'. They deal with the disappointment and immediately look for ways to improve their performance. If life gives you lemons, and you believe you can cope with a difficult situation, then you only need to make lemonade if you like lemonade.[5]

High frustration tolerance then, or the 'I Can Copes', or more specifically, 'I can cope with this difficult, demanding, challenging thing', is how the tough get going when the going gets tough. It puts meat on the bones of 'whatever doesn't kill you makes you stronger'; and it also means that, while you can keep the sick sense of humour and the weird coping strategies that you do enjoy, you can definitely ditch the ones that you don't, or the ones that are no longer serving you well.

And so, on to the final healthy belief, the fourth fix to the thoughts that fuck you up and the healthy equivalent to the pejorative put-down.

In the next chapter you are going to learn to accept yourself, perhaps even love yourself. And, not only yourself, but also other people; as well as life and the conditions contained within it.

And, if not love, then at least accept all people and all things as they are and drop a whole load of resentment and hatred as you do so . . .

---

[5] Actually, a lemon is a hybrid; it's a cross between a bitter orange and a citron. It didn't exist in nature, a human being made them. Therefore, life doesn't give you lemons, people do (or did, many years ago, when someone first thought, 'I wonder what I'll get if I cross "this" with "that"?'

Unconditional Acceptance

You either walk inside your story and own it, or you stand outside your story and hustle for your worthiness.

Brené Brown

In Rational Emotive Behaviour Therapy, the antithesis of the pejorative put-down is unconditional acceptance. Unconditional acceptance of the self, of other people and of life and all the conditions it contains. Intrinsic to this notion are two concepts: namely 'worth' and 'fallibility.' But, what does all this mean exactly? What is unconditional acceptance and how does it relate to worth and fallibility? Well, to explain, I'd first like to get all 'dictionary' about things.

Unconditional means 'not subject to any conditions' or 'complete and not limited in any way', while, in this context, acceptance means 'the process or fact of being received as adequate, valid or suitable'. Worth, meanwhile, means 'sufficiently good, important or interesting enough'. Finally, fallible means 'capable of making mistakes or of being wrong'.

When it comes to your beliefs about yourself, and other people or life conditions, then everyone and everything is complete and not limited in any way, adequate and valid, sufficiently good and yet capable of making mistakes, of being wrong and having failings.

I hope you can see where I'm going with this.

Every single human being on this planet is a worthwhile but fallible human being, and every single human being on this planet is a complex organism made up of many, many things; both the good and bad, the right and wrong, the successes and the failures and is an on-going story that will contain many, many more successes and failures to come.

If you fail your driving test, it simply means you failed your driving test. If you fail it five times, it only means you failed it five times. If you fail it a hundred times, it just means you probably can't do that thing, but not being able to do that thing does not make you a failure as a person.[1]

You are not a total failure, even if you fail many times at the same thing; you are a worthwhile but fallible human being. You are not a total loser, even if you are unlucky in love; you are a worthwhile but fallible human being. You are not a total idiot, even if you are not very clever in certain areas; you are a worthwhile, fallible human being. Your humanity is what makes you sufficiently good, important and interesting enough.

Your worth, then, is innate; you are born with it, and everyone else is too. Every human being is a fallible human being. Every single person on this planet had made mistakes, and they will make many more. So many mistakes: big ones, small ones and everything in between.

As your worth is innate, your 'stuff' does not add to your worth. Those ticks in the picture of you: getting things right,

_____

[1] Please don't offer me a lift home though.

your successes and your achievements do not add to your worth. Sure, they are nice things to get, they are feel-good moments in the story of your life, but they do not add to your worth one little bit.

By the same token, those crosses in the picture of you, all the getting it wrong you've done, the mistakes you've made and the people you've upset do not take away from your worth; it simply proves you're fallible. They won't be feel-good moments, and they can be downright disappointing, but your value as a human being does not need to take a knock.

When you use self-esteem as your yardstick, when you play its rating game, both your mood and your sense of self are tied to your achievements. Get it right and confidence and mood go up but get it wrong and both confidence and mood go down. You can overcompensate by only focusing on the successes or undercompensate by only focusing on the negatives. When you unconditionally accept yourself as a worthwhile and fallible human being, however, your confidence is more stable because your sense of self is more stable. When you get things right (yay!) your mood goes up, but your sense of self remains stable and, when you get things wrong (boo!), your mood dips, but again, your sense of self remains stable.

Basing your confidence on your worth means that your confidence levels and your sense of self are both stronger and more stable than when you base your confidence and your sense of self on your achievements.

Everyone deserves to feel good about themselves: and that includes you too. Self-worth comes from accepting yourself as you are, unconditionally, warts and all: good and bad, right and wrong, with all the success and all the failures that you have had, are having and will have to come. And happiness and positive self-talk comes from basing your confidence on your innate sense of self-worth. When you get things right, your mood will lift and when you get things wrong, your mood will drop, but your sense of self remains the same throughout.

You are a worthwhile, fallible human being, even when you fail at something, make a mistake or fuck up on a monumental level. Put paid to foolish notions such as 'a leopard can't change its spots' or 'once a cheater always a cheater'.[2]

Every single human being, no matter who they are or what they've done, is a worthwhile, fallible human being. Yes, they are. Every. Single. One. And it's at this point that people who are really, really determined to hate on themselves mention Hitler. They always mention Hitler.

'So, does that mean Hitler was a worthwhile, fallible human being too?' they ask, thinking they've outfoxed their REBT therapist. But, the answer is yes. Yes, he was. Ethically speaking, that's quite the tuppence to be spinning around upon, but allow me to explain.

I apologise for simplifying history but, early in his career, Adolf Hitler took a depressed Germany (unemployment was 15 per cent, people were homeless and starving) that, being a young nation, had yet to formalise a sense of 'identity'. A strong speaker, he motivated and galvanised the population

---

[2] A leopard can't change its spots, that much is true. It's part of their pigmentation and colouring but as an analogy for the human condition it's poppycock. People do change, people rehabilitate, they self-improve. And, for every cheater who cheated again, there's a cheater who did not.

and helped foster a sense of national pride. He was also allegedly a high achiever at school, kind to his mum, kind to animals and a vegetarian.

Also, whether you like it or not, his war effort facilitated a massive burst of scientific advancement and led to the creation of a variety of products that we still use today (including Volkswagen, the rocket engine and jet propulsion).[3] These are ticks in the picture of him.

However, he was a Nazi dictator, a bringer of war and, during the holocaust, responsible for the deaths of over six million human beings. These are very big crosses in the picture of him.

On a technicality, Hitler has good points and bad, achievements and failings. We need to believe in this, not for the dictators of the world, but for our justice system as, without it, there would be no rehabilitation. People are incarcerated with the hope that they can be rehabilitated and returned to so-called normal society. If they were not worthwhile, fallible human beings, how could that be possible?

However, some people, despite the ticks in the picture of them, have too many crosses, or crosses so severe that, for the good of society, they are locked away for life (or in some countries that still have the death penalty, that life is terminated). There were certainly enough crosses, and the crosses were big enough, that you could enact that penalty with Hitler were he alive, with just cause. But, we can neither deny nor invalidate the good he did.

---

[3] Jettas, Golfs, Passats, Polos, Herbie and cheap flights to Mallorca all exist because of Hitler.

However, you are not Hitler. And the people you are putting down are not Hitler. You, and they, are worthwhile, fallible human beings.

If you are using Hitler to justify hating on yourself or others, then ask yourself why. What have you ever done or what have they ever done to justify such hate, or deserve such a level of negative self-talk? The worst of us have good points and the best of us have bad points. And that is true of all of us.

Still don't believe me about worth? Then let's talk about children.

Do you have any? Let's say you do. Let's say one of them comes home and says, 'Mummy/Daddy/primary caregiver, I'm a total failure, my grades are rubbish right across the board, my friends have turned against me, I am a complete weirdo and therefore am completely useless.' Are you going to agree with them? Are you going to say, 'Yes, honey. Yes, you are,'? I'm really hoping that the answer you give is 'no'. It's certainly been a no every time I've used the analogy in the therapy room.

No, you're not going to agree with them. You are a good parent and/or primary caregiver, and you are going to teach them that they are perfectly fine just as they are. You will say that these things are but disappointments and, more importantly, that these disappointments do not define them; that today's failures can become tomorrow's successes if only they accept themselves and believe in themselves.

To put it another way, do you think your child, or your best friend's child, or any child for that matter, has more worth if they get things right and less worth if they get things wrong? If you can't empathise with children, perhaps it's your best friend. Would you agree with them if they espoused the belief that they were useless and worthless because of a current run of bad luck? Would their value to you go up and down depending on what they did and did not do, or on what they had achieved or failed at? No, of course not. You might want to take a look at your friendship skills if you do.[4]

When applied to a child or friend, you can see clearly that worth is innate. So, whether you like it or not, whether you believe it or not, this also applies to you. And, by definition it also applies to the people you don't like, and to all the people who you are currently pissed off with.

You are a human being, one of over seven billion human beings on this planet. And like every human being, you are born, you live and you die. You have no choice over the first or the last bit but, as far as the part in the middle goes, as you travel through this crazy thing called life, you get it right sometimes and you get it wrong sometimes, you achieve some things and you fail at others, you have things you are proud of and you have things you really want swept under the carpet and never, ever discussed again. Just like everyone else. In that we are all equal. We have different skills, different aptitudes, different stations in life, and different socio-economic statuses; but we are all a complex amalgamation of every single thing, good and bad and right and wrong, we have ever done and everything we will ever do going forwards.

---

[4] And, if you can't empathise with friends, I'm going to use puppies.

Your successes do not add to your worth and your failures do not detract from your worth. Your worth is innate. And REBT asks that you base your confidence on that.

You could, as invited earlier, complete the Herculean task of noting down absolutely every thing about you, every single tick and every single cross. But, by the end of it, you would only discover that, while you can (as Dr Hauck said) rate every conceivable thing, you cannot actually rate yourself totally as one thing or another. All you are left with then is unconditional acceptance of yourself as you currently are.

This doesn't mean you cannot change, because people do. It doesn't mean that failings cannot become successes, because they can. Sometimes. But, not always. As the very famous saying goes, 'Grant me the serenity to accept the things I cannot change, the courage to change the things I can and the wisdom to know the difference.'[5]

Some therapies do indeed advocate self-esteem. So, if you're lacking in confidence, they set homework experiments that ask you to go out and achieve something, to get something right. And, while I'm not knocking that as a strategy, there is an inherent risk. You are not going to fare well if you fail at your first task. Accepting yourself as that worthwhile, fallible human being is the more elegant solution. It could still allow you to go out and achieve something, but it wouldn't go so pear-shaped if you didn't achieve the thing that you wanted to achieve.

---

[5] The Serenity Prayer by Reinhold Niebuhr which, over time, has been secularized and non-secularized, depending on spiritual and religious leanings or lack thereof, and even adopted by Alcoholics Anonymous (AA) and other 12-step programmes.

In summary then, you are not Hitler, and the people you are putting down are equally not genocidal maniacs who need to be locked up for the common good.[6]

If you can accept your friends, your family, your work colleagues and the people around you as worthwhile, fallible human beings, then this concept also applies to you and to the people you are dissing.

To believe that you are not a failure, or useless, or rubbish or worthless, even if you don't get the thing that you want but, instead, are a worthwhile fallible human being is true. If you can evidence success, even if it's just one thing (which is incredibly simplistic) then you are not those things. We can prove that you are fallible because you get things wrong, you are a flawed human being.

Fallibility, you see, is built in and is fundamental to the notion of a human being because, you get things wrong. You also have psychological flaws (some people are too meek for their liking, while others are too bossy; some are prone to anxiety and others to depression). You also have physiological flaws (some of you go bald, some of you go grey prematurely, some people are prone to arthritis and others to heart disease). Fallibility is built in to all systems, including the human system.

Give up the rating game, a life of meaning does not necessarily mean a life of achieving. Another favourite quote of mine is this one by the philosopher Alan Wilson Watts: 'The meaning of life is just to be alive. It is so plain and so obvious and so simple. And yet, everybody rushes around in a great

---

[6] At least, I hope not.

panic, as if it were necessary to achieve something beyond themselves.'

Wise words indeed, but we're not done yet; let's back this up with some of that objectivity and rationality. Let us dispute these healthy beliefs.

Don't Forget Disputing

You are not a failure, or worthless, or useless, or no good, even if you don't get the thing you want, even if other people say you are. You are a worthwhile, fallible human being is totally true. If you can display so much as one success, one achievement, one accomplishment (which, let's face it, is a little simplistic), then you have all the proof you need to invalidate the useless/worthless/rubbish part of that statement. It's also true that you can get things wrong, that you have failed at things, that you have flaws, so the fallible bit is also true. Finally, if you are a human being then it is also true that you have innate worth as that human being.

You can rate individual aspects of the self, you can say I am great at English but rubbish at maths. But, being rubbish at maths is not the same thing as being rubbish as a person. Therefore, logically, you can only be a worthwhile fallible human being (and rubbish at maths being one of your failings).[7]

And finally, to believe this is helpful. You will still have an emotional reaction as you suffer those slings and arrows of outrageous fortune. So, if you accomplish something, or achieve something, you will feel excitement and a flush of

---

[7] If maths is important to you that is.

pride. If you fail at something, if you do not achieve what you set out to achieve, then you will feel a measure of disappointment. You may feel down, but not out. Getting things right and wrong will still affect your mood, but it no longer affects your sense of self. It no longer dents your confidence.

There is no greater evidence of this than the Olympic athlete who trains hard for four years to achieve a specific thing. Let's face it, there is really only one winner: it's the one that gets the Gold medal. But, even if you accept Silver or Bronze as a win, then there are all those who did not win either. And then, after the race, the event or the competition, the journalists round on the winners. 'How do you feel?' they ask. 'I feel great; yay me,' the winning athlete replies. But, the journalists also point their microphones and their cameras at the losers. And they're merciless. 'You lost,' they say. 'How do you feel?' they ask. And the losers do not say, 'Well, I feel shit. That's four years of my life down the drain. I have failed myself, and my country.' Well, not often at any rate. More often they say something along the lines of, 'Well, that was disappointing, but I'm going to sit down with my coach, look at the replay and see what I can do better next time.'

When you accept yourself unconditionally, as a worthwhile and fallible human being, there are no failures, only opportunities to learn.

This style of thinking also applies to others. So, when it came to my little problem, I think 'other people are not idiots; even if they get in my way, they are worthwhile and fallible human beings'. This belief was true, because they all had lives; they were all complex amalgams of every little thing, good and bad and right and wrong. I could guess that they had skills and aptitudes, even if I did not know them. People loved them. There were ticks in any picture of them I could care to build. However, I could most definitely evidence walking in to me and tripping over me as a failing on their part, so that part was covered too. And, finally, as human beings they all had worth because every human being does.

To believe that they were not complete idiots, even though they were actually getting in my way, was rational; to believe them worthwhile and fallible while they did so was equally rational, therefore one statement logically followed from the other.

And, this belief helped me. It allowed me to humanise rather than dehumanise; and to accept that we were all human beings together, simply doing our best to cope with a very crowded environment. No anger needed.

This concept of unconditional acceptance applies to the world and everything it contains. The world is very complex; it's got good things in it (such as puppies) and bad things in it (such as Ebola). So, it's not a complete write-off, it too is far too complex to completely write off. The world, then, is worthy in and of itself, but also fallible too.

Take my client who believed their life was total shit. The healthy version of this is 'No! My life is not total shit, even though it feels like it; my life is a worthwhile and fallible thing'. And this could be backed up with evidence (puppies and Ebola certainly, but also her specific successes and mistakes), could be looked at logically and could most definitely be viewed as helpful. It certainly helped this particular client out of her depression.

If you are indeed a project manager with a bit of a thing for perfection, you are not an abject failure if the project goes awry, the team you manage are not total <insert expletives here> just because they haven't completed things to your exacting standards and the project isn't a complete fail just because it didn't turn out exactly the way you wanted it to. You can dispute all three versions of this unconditional acceptance belief and prove them to be true, demonstrate their logic and show how they could help you.

How much better would you feel if you loved yourself, not in an egotistical way but in a nice way, the way you love a friend or family member? And if not love, then at least like and accept just as you are? How much easier would your life be if you focused on your assets rather than your detriments? How much more positive would you and others feel if you, equally, focused on their assets and good points as opposed to the bad. And, how would you feel if you focused on the good bits about life rather than the bad?

That's the power of unconditional acceptance, and it's so powerful that, over the years, it has helped many self-haters to become so appreciative of their lives that they've literally cried tears of joy.

Wouldn't you like to do that about yourself and your life?

The Four Thoughts That Don't F*ck You Up: A Summary

Thankfully for you, for your sanity and for your sense of self-preservation, every single one of the four unhealthy beliefs mentioned in this book has a healthy, rational equivalent, a 'fix' that will help you to think, feel and act more roundly, more rationally and more robustly in the face of adversity.

First up are the **Flexible Preferences** (where you state what you would like to have, but also accept that you don't have to have it); this is followed by **Perspectives** (also known as anti-awfulising, which is a more rational rating of the badness of you not getting what you want); then the **I Can Copes** (also known as high frustration tolerance, where you accept that not getting what you want is frustrating, but that you can deal with the frustration without dying or evaporating in a puff of exasperation), and finally, we have **Unconditional Acceptance** (of the self, of others and of life conditions). This is a more rational rating of people and things.

The important thing to note about your healthy beliefs is that they may not necessarily promote positivity. Neither do they necessarily promote neutrality. We are aiming for rationality. We are moving from an unhealthy negative emotion (one that controls you) to a healthy negative emotion (one that you control). Both the unhealthy and the healthy emotions contain the word 'negative'. REBT doesn't try and turn you into an emotionless robot that doesn't care when life doesn't go your way. It wants you to be human, it wants you to emote, but it wants you to emote appropriately; it wants you to emote in ways that are beneficial rather than detrimental to your mental health. This is what your healthy beliefs will do.

Understanding this is one thing, but believing it is another. Reading this book and going 'a-ha' is one thing, but actually putting it into practice and effecting a shift in the way you think, feel and act is another. As the old saying goes:

'knowledge is knowing a tomato is a fruit, but wisdom is knowing not to put it in a fruit salad'.

It may be that, as a result of reading the first two parts of this book, you've already had one or two epiphanies and have started to look at life, or certain situations, in a whole new light and to some beneficial effect.

More likely, however, is that you've noted that you hold these unhealthy beliefs and have even began identifying some of your demands, dramas, I can't copes and put-downs and written them down, which is great, because now you're going to learn how to work on them.

In Part Three of this book, you are going to take what you've learnt thus far, build on it and put it into practice. You are going to take your knowledge and distil it into wisdom.

Step-by-step and week-by-week, over the next six weeks you are going to learn more about the REBT ethos. You're going to pick a problem and break it down into its component parts. Next, you're going to identify the beliefs that give you a specific reaction in the face of a particular situation, then deconstruct them and think more rationally about them. After that you will be developing an emotional and behavioural shift. You will not only know what to say, but also believe what you are saying, so that you can effect a lasting change.

First things first though, let's put these unhealthy and healthy beliefs into a coherent strategy.

It's time to discuss the full philosophy and structure of REBT.

PART THREE

REWIRE HOW YOU THINK IN SIX WEEKS WITH RATIONAL EMOTIVE BEHAVIOUR THERAPY

Week One
REBT: A Cunning Plan

It's not what happens to you but how you react to it that matters.

Epictetus

I studied a year-long diploma that was based on REBT and then followed that up with a two-year MSc on the subject, so there's way more to this therapy that just four unhealthy beliefs and their more helpful equivalents. REBT has a philosophy, a framework and a plan to follow. It contains tools to help you challenge your beliefs. It can not only help you change the way you look at life in general, but also help you work on very specific emotional and behavioural problems. And working on one such specific problem is what you are going to be doing over the next six weeks and with the next six chapters.

Earlier in this book, I mentioned that Activating events (A) trigger Beliefs (B) that cause Consequences (C). I also mentioned that we Dispute (D) or challenge those beliefs to bring about an Effective (E) rational outlook to that original activating event. This is known, for very obvious reasons, as the ABCDE model of psychological health, and we will be exploring it in a little more detail shortly. Essentially, what it means is: there's a thing and there's always a reaction to the thing but, between the thing and the reaction, there's always a thought process involved.

That thought process, according to REBT, will always include a demand and then any one or more of the following: a drama (awfulising), or an I can't cope (low frustration tolerance) and/ or a put-down (a self-, other- or world-damning belief).

Over the next few chapters, and the next few weeks, you're going to learn how to pick a problem and work on it according to REBT's ABCDE model. You will learn how to identify which of the four thoughts you hold in the face of a particular problem, and then formulate the healthy equivalents to those thoughts. After that, you'll be engaging in a series of exercises that will help weaken your conviction in your unhealthy beliefs while, at the same time, build and strengthen a conviction in your healthy beliefs. Bit by bit, we will be effecting a shift from one way of thinking (unhealthy) to another way of thinking (healthy).

Before we get down to the nitty-gritty of what that means and entails, please allow me to lay down a few foundation stones.

The philosophy of REBT and the philosophy of this book are one and the same: that it's not the events in life that disturb you, but what you tell yourself about those events that causes problems.

That particular nugget of wisdom, and the quote at the beginning of this chapter, is based on the teachings of Stoic philosophy and, especially, the teachings of one Greek Stoic philosopher in particular. His name was Epictetus (55–135AD), and he even has a page on Wikipedia.

So, if you're thinking, feeling and acting in a way that you don't like, but don't seem to be able to change, it's not because of the 'thing', it's down to what you are telling yourself about the 'thing'. Change what it is that you tell yourself about that 'thing' and you get to change how you think, how you feel and how you act. This means that nobody and nothing makes you angry, anxious or depressed and nobody and nothing drives you to drink, drugs or distraction.[1]

Now, we're not saying that when stuff happens, it doesn't have an influence, because it does. But, it is only an influence. And yes, the more negative or challenging a situation is, the more of an influence it will be. But still: only an influence.

Even in the face of the most difficult and demanding of circumstances, you can still remain in control, or regain control if you think you've lost it, by looking at what you are telling yourself about that difficult and demanding thing.

As Captain Jack Sparrow once famously said, 'The problem is not the problem. The problem is your attitude about the problem.'

Don't believe me? Then, allow me to elaborate.

The General Principle of Emotional Responsibility

Let's say I get fired from my job and I spend the next few weeks and months telling myself, 'How dare they do that to

---

[1] Or doughnuts.

me? They must not get away with this, the rotten so-and-sos, I will get them if it's the very last thing I do!'

Chances are, I'm going to be (and am going to come across as) a very angry man indeed. I will be obsessed, consumed even. I will become one of those people who just aren't able to let things go.

But, what if I'm walking around telling myself, 'Oh no! They should not have done this to me, this is just terrible. How will I pay the rent? How will I pay my bills? I'm going to lose everything! I'll be destitute and homeless!'

Now, instead of being consumed by anger, I'm going to be consumed with anxiety, stricken with panic, frantically imagining a series of catastrophic events unfolding.

However, if I am walking around telling myself, 'That's it, game over, I'm no good for anything else. I'll never get another job, it's hopeless, I might as well give up now,' then, instead of feeling angry, or anxious, I'm going to be pretty depressed. I will feel helpless, hopeless and hard done by. I will probably retreat to my bedroom and stay there.

Anger, anxiety and depression are emotions that aren't particularly helpful, as I'll probably be too disturbed and dysfunctional to do anything constructive about my situation. Angry people rant, anxious people worry and depressed people hide away, and none of these things will help them deal with being fired in a helpful fashion.

But, what if I'm walking around thinking, 'Oh crap, I wasn't expecting that. I wish that hadn't happened, but it did; it will make life a little challenging, but I'll get through it, I always do. I've got skills, I'll probably find a better job with better prospects.' What will I feel then?

I'll most likely feel disappointed, but optimistic; frustrated but empowered and down, but not out. More importantly, I will be in a much better frame of mind to go out and do something constructive about my work-related situation.

Now, in each of the examples above, the situation was the same (being fired from my job). But, I could feel angry, anxious, depressed or even optimistic about being fired from my job, depending on what it was I told myself about being fired from the job.

And that is what Epictetus meant, all those years ago: *'It is not the events in life that disturb you; it's what you tell yourself about those events that disturbs you.'*

So, all human beings (by and large) are responsible for how they think, how they feel and how they act by the beliefs they hold in the face of any given situation – this is the General Principle of Emotional Responsibility.[2]

A Little Bit About Blame

Some people don't like the idea of the General Principle of Emotional Responsibility. They think they're being told that it's 'all their fault,' and that they are to blame for the way they are.

---

[2] This principle contains the caveat 'by and large'. As mentioned earlier, some people have clinical conditions (such as unipolar or bipolar depression). This is not a result of their beliefs, but down to various other factors, including brain chemistry. However, people with clinical conditions tend to develop very unhealthy beliefs about their unavoidable conditions that disturb them even further still.

More than a fair few people have fled my consulting room over the years, denouncing me as evil incarnate for even daring to suggest that their emotional and behavioural problems (and on one painful, but memorable occasion, their cancer diagnosis) were their fault (which I wasn't even slightly suggesting).

There's a whole realm of difference between blame and responsibility and one that, sadly, some people just don't seem to get.

Let's say that you're shopping in a supermarket and in aisles one and two you see and hear both a parent and a small child. In both aisles, the child is throwing an unholy tantrum of biblical proportions.

The parent in aisle one is admonishing their child: 'Oh my god, you're so stupid; you're so embarrassing. I am ashamed of you. Shut up! Just you stop this right now. Why are you so horrible?'

What is this child going to grow up thinking? What will it believe about itself? And, more importantly, will this child ever learn to take responsibility for its actions?

The parent in aisle two is also admonishing their child with equal frustration, but in a slightly different way. They're asking their child: 'Why are you behaving like this? Why are you behaving so badly? We both know you are better than this, so you tell me right now missy/mister/mx <delete where applicable>, why are you behaving so badly?'

Now, this is a small child the parent is dealing with here, so all they are likely to get is a shoulder shrug and a monotone mumble, 'I don't know.' But, that's not the point. The point is this: what will this child grow up thinking? What will it believe about itself? Will it be more likely or less likely to take responsibility for its actions than the child in aisle one? Why is that?

To be *responsible* is to be answerable or accountable for your actions. To be at *fault* is to believe yourself a failure for a wrongful act, that you are to be *blamed* for something.

Blame implies fault and, when it comes to how you deal with the stresses and strains of life, no one is at fault. There are only actions and reactions, and the responsibility for both. People at fault usually also go on and look for something else or someone else to blame for their wrongdoing. That way, they don't actually have to do anything about it.

It is not your fault that you are anxious, or depressed; it's not your fault that you've turned to alcohol or doughnuts as a coping strategy. But, if you blame yourself, you will feel at fault. More importantly, if you feel at fault, you will be less likely to take any responsibility for it; if you don't take responsibility for it, you won't be in a place where you feel like you can do anything about it. Instead, you'll feel stuck: stuck with who you are and how you are and with what you've got. Forever.

But, you are not responsible for other people, or how they behave, and you are not always entirely responsible for what life throws at you. What you are responsible for, however, is how you think and how you feel and how you act in the face of these things. Your thoughts are your responsibility. This is an empowering thing. Nothing else needs to change in order for you to change. Change is in your hands. Well, in your head. It was there all along.

AC Language Versus ABC Language

Take the 'Activating events trigger Beliefs that cause Consequences' ABC thing outlined at the beginning of this chapter – most people actually go through life talking what we call 'AC' language. They make the event responsible for how they feel. They say things like 'dogs scare me' or 'my boss makes me anxious' or 'what Maureen said about Our Sharon really makes my blood boil'. But, that's not how it works, that's not what is actually going on.

It feels true, because the process is instantaneous. Something happens and you have an emotional reaction to it. Plus, says your mind, if Maureen hadn't said that thing about Your Sharon, you would feel okay; if your boss was nicer, you wouldn't feel so anxious around them, and an absence of dogs clearly equals an absence of fear. To your mind, it's an emotional and behavioural cut-and-dried fact of life: if it hadn't have happened, you wouldn't feel the way you feel, right?

Wrong.

Because, instantly and unconsciously upon the event; you will have had a belief about that situation that triggered the reaction. So, when you see a dog, you tell yourself something that scares you; whenever you deal with your boss, you tell yourself something that makes you anxious; whatever it was what Maureen said about Your Sharon, you are telling yourself something that makes your blood boil.

REBT hones in on all those 'somethings'. It identifies them, it drags them up from the dark recesses of your mind and out into the cold light of day and then it challenges them. You might not know what yours are, not yet at any rate, but I'm hoping that several possibilities have sprung to mind as you read Parts One and Two of this book. If not, you can start thinking about them right now.

So, from now on, instead of saying, 'Blah, blah, blah makes me feel like so-and-so,' why not stop and think? Ask yourself instead, 'What am I telling myself about this thing that is making me feel this way?' It's the first step on the road to rational thinking.

These specific belief systems – about dogs, about your boss, about what Maureen said about Your Sharon, about anything and anyone that disturbs you –bring me to the next principle (if you accept the first principle that you are responsible, that is). It's your unhealthy beliefs that disturb you: it's your dogmatic demands, your dramas, your I can't copes and your put-downs that really disturb you.

The Specific Principle of Emotional Responsibility

As you go through this book and put it into practice, it will help you deal with life in general in a whole new way. Philosophically speaking, it's an excellent guide to rational living. Hopefully, you will have already begun to notice this. Therapeutically speaking, however, it is also excellent at helping you deal with specific emotional and behavioural problems.

Because (quite often), there are specific situations and there are specific reactions to those situations. Anger, for instance, is a specific reaction to something you find annoying; while anxiety is a specific reaction to something you find worrying. However, between the situation and the reaction there will be a specific belief system about that specific situation giving you that specific reaction.

REBT zeroes in on your specific anxiety- or anger- or depression-causing beliefs and seeks to change them. It makes a distinction between irrational beliefs (that do not help you in any given situation) and rational beliefs (which do).

So the four thoughts that fuck you up are four specific beliefs or patterns of thought, held in specific situations, that lead to a particular kind of emotional and behavioural reaction. To highlight exactly how they disturb you, I want to turn that thing about punctuality into a story, told in four parts, that will effectively communicate what REBT is all about.[3]

It's not for nothing that I've made timekeeping a thread that runs throughout the chapters on both the unhealthy and the healthy beliefs. As I've already mentioned, some people have a 'bit of a thing' for punctuality and some don't.[4] If you are, indeed, a person with a penchant for punctuality then, as you consider the following scenarios, this next bit is very important: *I don't want you to think like you, I want you to think like the person that holds the beliefs outlined in each scenario.*

With me so far? Good.

---

[3] The original version of this, developed by Albert Ellis, was called 'The Money Model' and involved beliefs about cold hard cash rather than time-keeping. Professor Windy Dryden later translated that model into English (i.e., he changed it from dollars to pounds). You can even find a version of it being practiced on YouTube. This is my own take on that model.

[4] Some people couldn't turn up on time to save their lives, whilst some don't even know what 'on time' means. And that's okay, for them. REBT can definitely help both the punctual, the sort-of-punctual and the very, very unpunctual get along in a much more harmonious fashion.

REBT in Relation to Punctuality

Part One

Imagine that you are on a train on your way to a very important appointment. I also want you to imagine that you have 'a bit of a thing' for punctuality. You have a belief about your punctuality, and your belief is this:

I prefer to be on time for everything, but I know I don't have to be. I don't like it when I'm not on time for everything, for me it's a bad thing; but it's not awful, or the end of the world, or anything like that.

Now your train gets delayed, badly, and you realise you are not going to make your appointment. The important question here is: how are you going to feel about that delay when your belief is 'I prefer to be on time for everything, but I know I don't have to be. It's bad when I am not on time for everything but it is not awful'? How are you going to behave with that belief?

You might be a little frustrated, or worried, but it wouldn't be any more than that. You won't like the fact that you have been delayed, but you will be able to deal with it. You might phone ahead to notify someone, or to rearrange the appointment but, other than that, you will, in all likelihood, just sit there and accept the delay as something beyond your control.

So far, so rational . . .

Part Two

I want you to imagine now that you are still on a train and that you are still on your way to that very important appointment. I also want you to imagine that you still have 'a bit of a thing' for punctuality. However, this time, you have a very different belief about your punctuality and, this time, your belief is:

Hell no! I must be on time for everything! I must, I must; I must! That's me! That's my thing! And if I don't get it, it is awful, it is like the end of the world to me!

Again your train gets delayed, badly, and again you realise you are not going to make your appointment. The important question now is, how are you going to feel about the delay with the belief 'I must be on time for everything and it is awful when I am not on time for everything'? How are you going to behave with this belief?

My guess is that you are going to be very angry, or very anxious, or both. You might blame yourself for not getting an earlier train, you might blame the on-board services manager or the entire franchise as a whole; you could possibly even shout and complain. You might phone ahead, but it would be a very different conversation than the one in the previous scenario. I doubt very much that you would sit there and calmly accept the delay.

So, the point you need to take from this so far is that, when faced with the same situation, two very different beliefs will give you two very different emotional and behavioural outcomes.

Now, I want to take the stressed, angry and/or anxious version of you a bit further.

Part Three

So, there you are: you're still on the train, you still hold the belief that you 'must be on time for everything, it is awful when you are not', and you are still delayed. You are stressed and angry and/or anxious. But then, the driver makes an announcement. He apologises for the delay, says he's going to speed the train up as much as possible, miss out a few of those little stations that no one really gets off at anyway, and get everyone to their destination on time.

This includes you. So the driver has just said he will get you there on time. Guaranteed it, even. Almost.

The important question here is this: how do you feel about being on time when your belief is 'I must be on time for everything, it is awful when I am not'?

You're going to feel relieved, right? Crisis averted, problem over, everything literally back on track? Phew!

Part Four

Now, the final part of the model is this. You're still on the train. You're still on your way to that oh-so-important appointment, and you still hold the belief that you 'must be on time for everything and it is awful when you are not'. You were delayed, but then the driver promised to get you there on time, so you felt relieved.

However, with the belief 'I must be on time for everything and it is awful when I'm not,' what one thing could happen to have you back to stressed and angry or anxious again? That's right: any other kind of delay.

The train only has to slow down a little bit, or stop at a platform too long for your liking, or come to a halt between stations and there you are right back to stressed out again.

And the point of that story was . . .

- So, REBT says that all human beings (yep, all of us, everywhere, all the time) are prone to emotional disturbance when they don't get what they *demand* they *must* have.
- REBT also says they are prone to further emotional disturbance, even when they do get what they *demand* they *must* have, because they can always lose it: it can be taken away and things can always change.
- It's only when they can assert a *preference,* but at the same time accept they *don't have to have* the thing that they prefer, that they can remain psychologically healthy.
- The difference between a demand and a preference means the difference between being unhealthily anxious or healthily concerned about not being on time for everything.

A little reminder . . .

- As human beings we have preferences for everything. We also have a tendency to take our preferences and turn them into demands.
- The stronger the preference, the more likely we are to turn them into demands.

Now, sometimes those demands are explicit, you can hear yourself, for example, literally shouting to the train manager (or to yourself), 'No, you don't understand! I have to be on time!' But, often, they're implicit, or unconscious. You don't know you're telling yourself that, you just know you're fuming because you're delayed. But, the demand is there (according to REBT), chugging away in the background and disturbing you.

So, that's the philosophy of REBT. But, it not only has a philosophy, it has a framework on which you can both hang and work on all of your problems and challenges.

It's the one I mentioned at both the beginning of this chapter and the beginning of this book.

The ABCDE Model of Psychological Health

The ABCDE model of psychological health is such an elegant way of looking at things that many other therapies have adopted this model since. Let's look at what those letters stand for in more detail.

A

This stands for the 'Activating event'. It's the situation, the problem, the thing you are disturbing yourself about. An activating event can be anything: a person, a situation, what someone said and so on. It can be something from the past, something from the present or something from the future. It could be something real or something imagined and it can be an internal event or an external event. Given such scope, anything then, can be an activating event:

public speaking, an exam, the effects of losing your job, that strange twinge in your side, that Thing You Did All Those Years Ago, what Maureen said about Your Sharon, absolutely anything.

In the four scenarios involving punctuality above, the delayed train was the activating event. More specifically, it was having 'a bit of a thing' for punctuality, or wanting to be on time for everything, that was the activating event. When you take an activating event, you need to identify the part of it that you find the most disturbing (this is known as the 'Critical A', but more of that later), because this will directly lead to the beliefs you need to work on.

B

The B stands for 'Beliefs'. There are unhealthy demands that can disturb you and healthy preferences that can help keep you rational based on the specific demand held in the face of that specific problem. The activating event will trigger a series of beliefs that causes consequences at C. If your beliefs are rational, your responses are rational, but if your beliefs are irrational, then your responses will, likewise, be irrational (i.e. unhelpful to you).

The punctuality story above included two of the unhealthy thoughts and two of the healthy thoughts, namely 'I must be on time for everything' and 'it is awful when I am not', and 'I prefer to be on time for everything, but I don't have to be' and 'it's bad when I'm not on time for everything, but it is not awful'.

C

This stands for the 'Consequences' of holding a particular belief. Consequences are you. They're your psychology; they're your thoughts, your feelings, your symptoms, your behaviours and your emotions. Anxiety will carry with it specific thoughts, feelings, behaviours and symptoms which will be very different from the thoughts, feelings, behaviours and symptoms of, say, anger. Every other disturbing thought you can have about a problem will be a result of a combination of the four thoughts that fuck you up.

So, for instance, when you have the belief 'I must not get anxious during my presentation, it would be awful if I did', then you are only increasing the likelihood that you will actually get anxious during your presentation. In fact, you might get so anxious beforehand that you refuse to do it, or try to do it but run out of the room in tears.

However, if you tell yourself 'I prefer not to get anxious during my presentation but there is no reason why I mustn't; it would be bad if I did that but it wouldn't be awful', you might be worried about your presentation in a nervous, excited way, but you won't get anxious, you won't avoid it, and you won't be found hiding in the toilet, weeping gently to yourself.[5]

D

The D stands for 'Disputing'. It is the process of challenging your beliefs (both the unhealthy and the healthy) over

---

[5] This has been known with anxiety.

and over again. Bit by bit, we are weakening the unhealthy ones and reinforcing the healthy beliefs; we are effecting a shift from one way of thinking to the other. When you can feel that shift take place, we know we have arrived at E. Disputing is where you have to put in the effort. The idea is that, whatever your goal, as you move towards it you challenge yourself, but you don't overwhelm yourself. However, the more effort you put in, the quicker you realise your goal.

E

This means you now have an 'Effective rational outlook' on that activating event. It is where you begin living life according to the rational beliefs and not the irrational ones. Using the timekeeping model from earlier, this is where you shift from becoming the angry or anxious person on the train to the calm but more accepting (shrug your shoulders and deal with it) type of person on the train.

In Summary

So, in this book you are going to learn how to take a problem or situation that you are disturbing yourself about and put it at A as an activating event.

You will then take that A and use it to work out what thoughts, feelings and behaviours you are exhibiting at C. This, in turn, will allow you to identify the Critical A (the aspect of the problem/situation that disturbs you the most).

The Critical A will then be used to correctly assess your unhealthy beliefs at B.

From there you can work out what your healthy beliefs need to be in order for you to hold more functional thoughts, feelings, behaviours and emotions at C.

You will then be taught to challenge and weaken your unhealthy beliefs and challenge and strengthen your healthy beliefs using a variety of disputing techniques at D.

When you can put this into practice and begin living your life according to your healthy beliefs (don't worry, we can help you do that too) you make an emotional and behavioural shift at C.

When this happens, you will have arrived at E, which means that you will now have an effective rational outlook to your original problem.

So, just like The Jackson 5 sang all those years ago, it really is as easy as ABC. Although, in Rational Emotive Behaviour Therapy, we prefer the term 'elegant'.[6]

And that's more or less it for Week One. Except for your homework. Homework is a big part of REBT. We don't mean homework like when you were at school. You won't be chained to your desk for an hour-and-a-half each night and you can eat your dinner if you don't do it. If you were to devote 15 to 20 minutes of your day, four or five days of the week to the homework set at the end of each week, that would be plenty. There, that doesn't sound too bad, does it?

---

[6] An elegant solution is preferable to a simple solution. And, by elegant, we mean pleasingly ingenious.

And, if you don't like the word 'homework', because, let's face it, it can remind you of school (and not everybody liked school, did they?), then you can call it an assignment, or even a project. One client of mine, who didn't like any of those terms, simply called it 'Stuff to Do'.

For those of you who don't like defacing books, this is where you need to turn to the notepad I mentioned buying. Or, you can download forms from my website: www.danielfryer.com.

Stuff to Do for Week One

- Read through the story about timekeeping a few times, as well as the ABCDE model and what each letter represents. You're not going to be tested on it or anything, but it explains everything that REBT is about, so the more familiar you are with it, the better equipped you will be going forwards.
- Have a go at explaining REBT to someone else using the story about timekeeping if you would like to. Sometimes, our nearest and dearest can throw up quite valuable insights, either about themselves or about you when you do so. 'OMG!' they exclaim, 'I do that then and you do that there.'

Before you turn to the Week Two chapter, answer the following reflective questions.

Reflective Questions

- What is this chapter about?
- Can you relate this model to you and your stuff; to any of your disturbances; to any of your anxieties, or depressions or outbursts, or simply to your life in general?
- Have you had any insights or 'light bulb' moments as a result of reading through and reflecting on the timekeeping example and the ABCDE model in the past week?

Week Two

How to Pick and Pick Apart a Problem

We don't see things as they are, we seem them as we are.

Anaïs Nin

So, there's going to be a lot going on in this chapter. It's probably the biggest chapter of the book. Sorry about that. Can't be helped. But, I will break it down into bite-sized chunks.[1]

Do feel free to take your time, and spread things out over the course of the day or the week.

First of all you're going to pick a problem to work on, then identify the correct unhealthy emotion held in the face of that problem. Next, you're going to identify the aspect of the problem that disturbs you the most and, from there, identify all of the unhealthy beliefs that you hold in the face of that

---

[1] Not that REBT is edible. Ewww.

problem. Finally, you will formulate the healthy equivalents to those beliefs. That doesn't sound like too much now does it?

Also, you need a goal in mind. Goals are very important in REBT. Therapeutically, what do you want to happen when you work on your problem? Emotionally and behaviourally, what is it that you want to achieve?

For instance, your goal might be to control the anxiety you feel when speaking in public, or to control your anger at home. Maybe you want to deal with your relationship jealousy, or stop feeling depressed about the loss of your job, and so on. In essence, this chapter is all about picking an Activating event at A, assessing the correct emotional Consequence at C in the face of that event, and then formulating your Beliefs at B.

Again, if you don't want to write in this book, or if you're reading this on a Kindle then, you might want to turn to your notebook and pen.

How to Pick a Problem

Most people, when they come to therapy, try to tell their entire life story. At least, in the first session they do. The therapist makes notes, and tries to find out as much as they can, not only about 'the problem', but all the other issues leading up to and impacting upon the problem. They are trying to understand their client as much as possible and, as soon as the client starts talking, the REBT therapist's mind is whirring, sifting through the information, formulating hypotheses and potential consequences and possible beliefs. This can easily take up half the session or more.

Some clients, however, come in with everything neatly summarised on a side or two of A4, a kind of *Potted History of Me*. People that do this usually take to REBT very well indeed.

Others, however, come in, sit down and literally say: 'I'm angry with my boss,' or 'I'm really anxious about performing,' or 'I have perfectionist issues.' And that's it. Not much else by way of information is given, and so we explore that specific issue in a little more detail.

I am hoping that, as you have made it this far, you already have a specific problem in mind. Maybe it's a work issue, or a relationship issue. Maybe it's the loss of something, or a problem with sitting exams and taking tests but, for now, the Activating event – the problem you would like to work on – only has to be defined as simply as that. And you can define the emotion just as simply, for the moment. So perhaps you're stressed at work, or angry with your partner, or depressed about that loss, or anxious about exams.

In the ABCDE model you are filling in the A and the C in the broadest of strokes. It might look like this:

A	C
Work	Stress
Partner	Anger
Loss of job	Depression
Exams	Anxiety

Maybe you want to come up with a list of problems; maybe the list above is your list of problems. But, and here is the important part, for the purposes of this book you need to select just one problem for now. Maybe the most pressing, or the most disturbing or, simply the one you would like to work on first.

For instance, as an example over the next few chapters, I'm going to use social anxiety as a case study, mainly because it's a very common problem.

Theo: A Case of Social Anxiety

Let's meet Theo, who came to see me because he did indeed have such a problem. Now, Theo was the sort of person that had already written things down on a piece of paper, which read: 'I get angry with my boss sometimes, I'm nervous in pretty much any and all social situations and some work situations, I'm not very confident in general and I also feel guilty because I let my friends down a lot.'

Top of that list for Theo, problem number one, was 'nervous in pretty much any and all social situations'.

Very broadly speaking, we have an Activating event at A and an emotional Consequence at C for this person:

A	C
Social Situations	Nervous

But, what does Theo mean by 'nervous', and is it an unhealthy kind of nervous or a healthy kind of nervous? In short, we need to look at the consequences in a little more detail.

Finding Your 'C'

In REBT there are eight unhealthy negative emotions and eight healthy negative emotions. That's it. The sum total of almost all human reactions to things literally boils down to one of these emotions, or a combination thereof.

Simply put, an unhealthy negative emotion is an inappropriate emotional reaction to a challenging event or situation, while a healthy negative emotion is an appropriate emotional reaction to the same challenging event or situation.

As I mentioned earlier, REBT isn't trying to promote positivity (although you may feel more positive) and it isn't trying to promote neutrality (although you may feel more neutral). It is, however, promoting rationality. And, sometimes, the most rational thing you can say is, 'Well, that sucks!' when something goes wrong. Sometimes, it's completely rational to feel a little concerned about the things that you find important, or very concerned about the things you find really important.

Let's say I have an exam coming up. If my belief is 'I must pass the exam and it will be awful if I don't', then I am going to make myself anxious about that up-and-coming exam. My revision will be more chaotic, my memory poor and my sleep disrupted. I will be more likely to perform poorly, or panic and not perform at all.

However, if I hold the belief 'I would prefer to pass my exam, but I know I don't have to pass it; it will be bad if I don't pass, but it won't be awful', I'm not going to become cocky or blasé about the exam, I will still care, because I prefer to pass. So, I will have an emotional reaction to the exam, but that emotion will be concern, worry or, even, nervous excitement. As a result, my revision and memory will both be improved, as will my sleep and I will be more likely to do well on the day of the exam.

So, let's look at the eight unhealthy negative emotions and their healthy counterparts in turn. Please bear in mind that this is a self-help book and no substitute for a good therapist, especially if you're dealing with a number of issues or are, emotionally, at the severe end of the spectrum or are dealing with a clinical condition. So, if after reading the following, which is the briefest of introductions to each emotion, you are finding it hard to pin down the emotion, or finding it hard to sift through a set of competing emotions, it would be best to put the book down, seek out the services of a professional, and come back to it at a later date.

The eight unhealthy emotions and their corresponding healthy negative emotions are:

Anxiety	Concern
Depression	Sadness
Anger	Annoyance
Unhealthy Jealousy	Healthy Jealousy
Unhealthy Envy	Healthy Envy
Guilt	Remorse
Hurt	Disappointment
Shame	Regret

Each unhealthy emotion has its own theme (or inference) and comes with typical thoughts and behaviours attached. The eight healthy negative emotions will also come with thoughts and behaviours typical to that particular emotion. But, the related thoughts and behaviours will be more reasonable, rational and appropriate. Unhealthy beliefs will always lead to unhealthy negative emotions and behaviours while, unsurprisingly, healthy beliefs will lead to healthy negative emotions and behaviours.

UNHEALTHY: ANXIETY

The theme (or inference) of anxiety is threat or danger. When you are unhealthily anxious you typically over-estimate the probability of that threat occurring and you under-estimate your ability to deal with it. You're also more likely to create even more negative or nightmarish threats in your mind and are more likely to find it hard to concentrate on the daily tasks of living (i.e. you are easily distracted). In terms of behaviour, anxious people will either avoid the thing they are anxious about, or tolerate it under extreme duress (i.e. with very obvious signs and symptoms of anxiety). They may tranquilise their feelings with alcohol or drugs (prescription or recreational), seek reassurance ('Am I alright? Am I alright? I am alright, aren't I?') or ward off the threat with superstitious behaviour.

HEALTHY: CONCERN

This is the healthy version of anxiety. It has the same theme, namely, a threat or danger. However, when people are healthily concerned (or worried), they don't over-estimate the probability of that threat occurring and they don't underestimate their ability to deal with it. They don't usually create even more negative and nightmarish threats or dramas in their mind and, despite there being something to worry about, are more able to concentrate on the daily tasks of living. As a result they will face up to the threat and/or danger and deal with it constructively (if and when it happens) and will even take constructive action to minimise the possibility of it occurring. There's no avoidance, no need to tranquilise and no desire to seek reassurance or engage in superstitious behaviour. Basically, if you're healthily concerned your attitude is one of, 'Okay, I will deal with this, even though I don't like it,' or, 'I will deal with this, if and when it happens.'[2]

UNHEALTHY: DEPRESSION

Anxiety looks forward, to the future, to things that haven't happened yet and probably won't happen at all. Depression looks backwards, to the past, to things that have happened and that most probably can't be changed. The theme (or inference) of depression is loss and failure (with implications for the future, because there is a teensy bit of forward projection). When you are unhealthily depressed you only

---

[2] Emphasis on the 'if'. When you are unhealthily anxious, you have already decided it will happen. When you are healthily concerned, 'when it happens' often becomes 'if it happens'.

see the negative aspects of that loss or failure, you have a tendency to dwell on all the other losses and failures you have ever experienced and, as a result, feel pretty helpless and hopeless. You decide that your future most definitely does not look bright. Depressed people withdraw from reinforcements (work, exercise, hobbies, friends and family and so on) and into themselves. They can create environments that are consistent with their feelings (letting their appearance go, letting household chores build up, etc.) and may attempt to terminate their feelings of depression in self-destructive ways (with alcohol, with prescription medication or recreational drugs and, even, in extreme cases, with suicide attempts).

HEALTHY: SADNESS

This is the healthy expression of depression and it is still sticking with the theme of loss and failure (with implications for the future). Because life does contain both losses and failures; sometimes, more than we would like. However, when you are healthily sad, although not a pleasant experience or emotion, you are able to see both the positive and negative aspects of that loss or failure, do not tend to dwell on other losses and failure and, as a result, although down, you don't feel helpless or hopeless. You can see a future, and that future does indeed look brighter than your present. You are able to talk about your feelings with others (friends and family and so on) and, although you may withdraw a little as you process that loss or failure, it's not long before you are engaging with life and all that it entails again (work, hobbies, socialising and the like).[3]

UNHEALTHY: ANGER

Anger is all about frustration, goal obstruction, rule-breaking and threats to our self-esteem. Life can be frustrating, our goals get thwarted and we all have personal rules that sometimes get broken, either by ourselves or by others. When we are unhealthily angry, we over-estimate the extent to which another person acted deliberately; or see malicious intent in the motives of others; we tend to assume a position of moral authority (I am absolutely right and you are absolutely wrong); we find it hard, if not impossible, to see the other person's, point of view, and may plot and, even, exact our revenge. Behaviour-wise, well, you know what angry people do: they may go on the attack physically or verbally (or both); or they may act in passive-aggressive ways ('I'm fine' they say, when actually, they're not, they just want you to work a little harder at finding out). They might displace their anger

---

[3] When you are clinically or severely depressed people try to tell you things such as, 'Cheer up, it's not that bad,' or, 'Have you tried not being depressed?' It's because they don't understand what depression feels like, they don't understand what it does. They've never had it, and so their only frame of reference is 'sadness'. The only way they could know what you were going through is if they had experienced it themselves. And if they had, they wouldn't be saying such things in the first place.

(by kicking the cat or slamming the door) or storm off in a huff (also known as withdrawing aggressively), and may even try to recruit other people against the person or people they are angry with.

HEALTHY: ANNOYANCE

Sticking with the same theme (or inference), namely frustration, goal obstruction, rule-breaking and threats to our self-esteem, because these things can and will occur, even when you are a perfectly rational person. However, here you do not over-estimate how deliberate the other person was; you are less likely to see malicious intent in their actions; you drop the moral absolutism (so it's less right-wrong and more shades-of-grey); are much more able to see things from their point of view, plus there's no skulking about and plotting your revenge. Annoyed people exhibit different behaviours. They're more able to let it go if it's not that important, or communicate their frustrations effectively if it is. They will assert themselves more effectively and request change from the person that frustrated them if they deem it necessary. That's *request* change, not demand change, because we don't like demands in REBT, do we? And an annoyed person will leave a situation calmly, once they have dealt with it to the best of their ability.[4]

---

[4] No cats get kicked, no doors get slammed and, when asked, nobody says, 'I'm fine,' unless they are actually fine.

UNHEALTHY: JEALOUSY

The theme here is 'concern for your relationship'. Normally, it involves your significant other, but there are other types of jealousy, such as sibling rivalry. With your relationship, there's a threat (usually involving another person). Here, you think your significant other has cheated, is cheating or will cheat or that some 'other' is making a move on them. When you are thinking irrationally, you see threats where none actually exist; can think that the end of your relationship is well and truly nigh; misconstrue your partner's conversations and behaviour as having romantic or sexual connotations; vividly imagine your other half up to all sorts and will go bat shit crazy if your partner even admits to fancying another person. The unhealthily jealous person typically seeks constant reassurance; will monitor their partner's actions and feelings; possibly search for evidence that they are involved with another (hello text checking and email hacking); try to restrict their partner's movements and activities; sulk, set tests and traps (for instance, getting someone to chat them up when they're out and then informing you of their response) and even retaliate for the presumed infidelity by, well, cheating themselves.

HEALTHY: JEALOUSY

This isn't the same as being secure in your relationship. Think of it as trust, tinged with a little nervousness. Because, again, we have the same theme here, namely 'concern for your relationship'. Maybe someone is interested in your man/woman/gender-fluid significant other. People don't stop being attractive to others, or finding others attractive, just because they're dating or married. However, you are more able to view your partner's interactions as harmless (even if they are flirting or being flirted with). 'It's just banter,' you conclude. You do not imagine them seeing someone else, and can accept (more or less with good grace) that your other half finds other people attractive. However, you do not see these attractions as a threat. Here, your partner is free to express their love for you, without your need for constant reassurance. You don't feel the need to monitor their whereabouts, thoughts, feelings or actions. No one is setting any honey traps, no one has to chime in every half hour by text just to be safe, and you won't go out and shag another just because your partner smiled at someone. There, isn't that nice?

UNHEALTHY: ENVY

Similar to, but different from, jealousy, envy's theme is that someone else has got something you desire very much, but don't yourself possess. Maybe it's a new promotion, the latest iPhone, an Aston Martin or a hot new romantic interest. When you are unhealthily envious, you have a tendency to insult and denigrate the value of the thing possessed or the person that possesses it, you try to convince yourself (unsuccessfully) that you are happy with your lot. You may plan how to acquire one yourself, regardless of need or use, or plot to deprive the other person of their treasured possession or think about how you could spoil it or destroy it. You may insult and denigrate the person or their possession and even try to take it away, or physically destroy it, so they don't actually have it anymore. Childish, I know.

HEALTHY: ENVY

Okay, so someone may very well have something you desire very much, but don't yourself possess. However, when you are on the healthy side of this particular emotion, you simply fess up and admit that you would like to have something like that; you do not try to convince yourself that you're happy with your lot when you're not; you can think about how to obtain one because you genuinely want one yourself; can allow the other person to have and enjoy the possession you desire, without you denigrating them or their thing; and, if you really want it, you will work towards getting one yourself. No one throws any wobblers, and nobody's toys get broken.[5]

UNHEALTHY: GUILT

Guilt is all about sin. There's the sin of commission (I did something I shouldn't have), and then, there's the sin of omission (I didn't do something I should have done). And,

---

[5] 'I'm so jealous,' you laugh, even though you mean envy, whilst congratulating them on their 'thing'.

right there, we're already in trouble, because both those sentences contain demands. We all have a moral code. Sometimes we violate it, either accidentally or deliberately, and sometimes we fail to live up to that code. These 'sins' can hurt the people we care about. However, when the beliefs and the emotion are unhealthy, the guilty party assumes that they have definitely committed the sin, assumes more personal responsibility than the situation warrants or deserves, assigns far less responsibility to the other party, does not consider any mitigating factors or put their behaviour into an overall context and thinks (or believes) that they will receive some form or retribution. And, what do the guilty do? Well, typically, they try to escape the pain of guilt in self-defeating ways, to beg forgiveness from the person they wronged and promise (unrealistically) that they will never, ever sin again, punish themselves (either physically or by depriving themselves of something), disclaim responsibility for the wrongdoing and reject any and all offers of forgiveness.

HEALTHY: REMORSE

Still with sin, because sometimes (moral code-wise) we do things we shouldn't have done, or don't do things we should have done, and then the people we care about get hurt. However, when your beliefs are healthy and the emotion you feel is remorse, things change. You're more likely to consider your behaviour in an overall context before deciding if you have actually sinned, tend to assume an appropriate level of personal responsibility, but also assign an appropriate level of responsibility to others. You also take the mitigating factors into account, put their behaviour into an overall context and do not think you will be receiving any retribution. That person will face up to the pain that comes with the sin; will ask for but not beg for forgiveness (and also accept such offers of forgiveness); understand their reasons behind the wrongdoing and act on it accordingly; atone for and make amends, and not try to excuse their behaviour.

UNHEALTHY: HURT

The theme of hurt is that someone has treated you badly when you didn't deserve it. This 'other' is usually significant (partners, friends, family members). When you are hurting this way, you over-estimate the unfairness of their behaviour; you believe that they don't care or are indifferent to your suffering; you feel alone, uncared for and misunderstood; and you tend to reflect on past hurts and expect the other person to make the first move in repairing the relationship and healing the hurt. Typically, the hurt person won't talk to the other person, preferring to shut down communication. However, they will sulk and make it very clear that they are upset, while not disclosing what it is they are upset about, they may even criticise or punish (indirectly, because they're not talking to them, remember?).

HEALTHY: DISAPPOINTMENT

Sticking with the same inference, someone has treated you badly and you didn't deserve it. They are 'significant.'

However, now you're healthy, you are more realistic about how unfair they have been, you see them as having acted badly rather than being uncaring or indifferent to your plight. You don't feel alone, or uncared for, or misunderstood, and you don't tend to dwell on past hurts. Also, you don't think the other person has to make the first move in healing the hurt. This way, you are able to communicate your feelings effectively and are able to influence them to act in a fairer way towards you.

UNHEALTHY: SHAME

And, so to shame, where you feel something shameful has been (or soon will be) revealed about either yourself, or the people you associate with (either by yourself or by others); where you feel you have acted in a way that falls short of your ideals or you believe others will either look down on you or shun you or the group you associate with. Quite a lot going on there, I'm sure you'll agree. When you are unhealthily ashamed you tend to over-estimate the 'shamefulness' of the information or gossip, while not only overestimating the degree to which people will be interested (or even notice, or care), but also the depth of their disapproval and the amount of time that this will all go on for. The shameful person will typically cut themselves off from other people, hide themselves away, try to save face by going on the attack, defend their self-esteem in self-defeating ways, and ignore any attempts by other people to restore social harmony.

HEALTHY: REGRET

And finally, to regret, where maybe something regrettable has been revealed about either yourself, or the people you associate with (either by yourself or by others); where you feel you have acted in a way that falls short of your ideals or you believe others will either look down on you or shun you or the group you associate with. However, with your healthy beliefs and healthy emotions, you are able to see yourself and the gossip in a compassionate and self-accepting way, are not only more realistic about how interested other people will be, but also about how much disapproval you will actually receive and how much time it will go on for. As a result, you continue to participate in social activities and you respond well to any attempts other people make at mediating and restoring social harmony. Which is really rather nice, for all concerned.

Consequences In a Nutshell

So, there you have it, the eight unhealthy negative emotions and their eight healthy counterparts. When it comes to picking one to work on: if you feel under threat and want to avoid something it's anxiety; if you feel like you've failed or suffered a loss and feel hopeless and helpless and want to hide away, it's depression; if you feel that someone has broken your unwritten rule and you want to give them a very loud piece of your mind, it's anger; if you're worried about your relationship and go crazy if they so much as talk to another person, it's unhealthy jealousy; if someone else has something you want and you resent them for it, it's unhealthy envy; if you feel that you have done something wrong and definitely deserve to be punished, it's guilt; however, if you feel someone else has done you wrong and you didn't deserve it, but you're going to sulk and expect them to make the first move, it's hurt. Finally, if you're, like, so embarrassed that you're hiding away from all your friends, it's shame.

Anxiety and depression are the number one and number two most common symptoms that people present with in therapy. When talking about depression here, I am talking about depression as an emotional problem, not a clinical condition – as a reaction to something specific, such as the loss of a job, a relationship or social status or, even, life itself.

Depression caused by life itself may seem like a vague, rather than a specific, thing, a philosophical conundrum rather than an activating event, but it can be a specific problem in itself.

Many years ago, when I was but a few months into practising professionally as a therapist, I had a client who asked me to help him with his depression. He was having trouble pinning down exactly what it was he was depressed about. And, because I was new to this, and because I had been taught to keep going until I had helped a person define something specific to work on, I kept barraging him with questions. Question after question until, in the end, and through a cloud of snot and tissues, he wailed, 'It's my life, my life is shit, it's just shit,' and began crying. And I realised that life was indeed the activating event and that the demand was 'my life should not be so shit'. And so, that is what we worked on.

What Do You Do If You Think Your Emotions Are Healthy?

Well, nothing really, except to maybe make yourself a nice cup of tea or coffee, and carry on reading this book as a point of interest only. This is a good thing. It means you're fine, your emotions are fine and you don't have any emotional problems to work on; it means that your reactions are healthy and appropriate reactions. Some people come to therapy with what they think are emotional problems and are surprised (sometimes pleasantly so) to discover that they are actually thinking, feeling and acting in healthy, constructive ways. It's perfectly okay to be worried (but not anxious) about your up-and-coming exam; it's rational to feel sad (but not depressed) about the break-up of a relationship or the loss of a job and it's perfectly acceptable to be annoyed or frustrated (but not angry) with someone's unacceptable behaviour. We don't want you to feel 'nothing' when life presents you with challenges and difficulties, because that would be weird. If your thoughts and behaviours are in line with the healthy negative expression of a particular emotion then all is well.

Next, we are going to assess the ABC in an ABCDE problem so having read through the list of emotions, if you already have a problem in mind and think that some of what you read applies to you, please make a note of it.

Assessing the 'A'

So, back to Theo. To find out what was going on with him, I wanted him to relate to me a specific example of being 'nervous' about a social situation. I asked him to give me one that was typical of the problem that he wanted to work on, and also an event that was either the most recent, the most memorable or the most vivid in his mind. I wanted the event that he was going to recall and retell to be as specific, memorable and vivid as possible because, that way, we get the disturbed juices flowing and will be more likely to discover what is going on. Theo told me this . . .

Theo's Activating event

'Well, it's the final thing that brought me here really. It was my friend Beth's birthday last month. I guess she's my best friend. She was throwing a party. She knows I have a problem with socialising but she really wanted me there and made me promise to go. Which I did but, as soon as I promised, I felt uneasy and, as the date approached, I got more and more anxious. Sometimes it was all I could think of, worry-ing about all the things that would go wrong; I'd forget what I was doing sometimes. The week leading up to the party was especially rough. It affected my sleep then, as the day arrived, I bottled it and cancelled. I didn't go. Then I felt really guilty for letting Beth down. She was so disappointed in me and that's when I decided to do something about it. I do this all the time, I always say I will go, kid myself that I might but know that I won't, then pull out, and feel guilty for letting someone down.'

From the above story it's clear that Theo has unhealthy anxiety about social events. Not only is the emotion getting in the way of the daily tasks of life (sometimes he forgets what he is doing, plus it affected his sleep), he also engaged in avoidance by not going to the party. Goal-wise, Theo's needs were very clear. He wanted to control his anxiety, to be able to socialise, attend parties and not let friends down.

So, Theo's ABC formulation is beginning to look like this:

A	C
Beth's party	Anxiety

Next, we needed to assess Theo's Activating event a little more thoroughly. Being too anxious to go to Beth's party isn't enough information to discover which of the four thoughts were fucking him up, or what they were specifically. There could be many aspects of socialising that he found disturbing and was getting anxious about, but one aspect would be the most disturbing of all, one aspect would provoke the most anxiety.

People tend to know themselves very well and you know yourself very well too, which is handy because, in a little while, I'm going to get you to sketch out a problem just like this. For now, I asked Theo to close his eyes and imagine the day of the party, and then asked, 'What did you find so anxiety provoking about going to Beth's party?' And it would be highly likely that Theo would be able to answer. He might have replied, 'Saying something wrong,' or, 'Not being liked' or, even, 'Being judged by the other people there.' Whatever answer he gave would be the aspect of the Activating event (Beth's party) that disturbed him the most. This is known as the Critical A. I'll repeat that, because it is important.

The Critical A is the aspect of the event that disturbs the most.

If Theo couldn't have given a succinct or definite answer, we could have come up with a list of all the things that he found anxiety provoking about going to Beth's party. And the list could have looked like this:

- Saying something wrong
- Not being liked
- Being judged by other people
- Having nothing to say
- Making a fool of myself
- People noticing my nerves
- People knowing that I am shy
- Being too shy to talk

Now we're getting somewhere. Now we understand what Theo is getting anxious about more clearly. All of the items on Theo's list are anxiety provoking and would create unhealthy beliefs. But, one of those items is the most anxiety provoking of all and would create the unhealthy beliefs we need to work on in order to literally get Theo to the party. When asked which item he found most anxiety provoking of all, Theo picked 'being judged by other people'. Ladies, gentlemen and variations thereupon, we now have a winner. And Theo's ABC formulation now looks like this:

A	C
Being judged by other people	Anxiety

Now it's your turn. I want you to write down a problem – an Activating Event – at A and, using the emotions discussed above as a guide, address a Consequence at C.

A	C
My activating event is:	My emotion is:

Now, I want you to take a specific example of the problem, just like Theo did, picking an example that is typical of the problem that you want to work on, but also an example that is either the most recent, the most memorable or the most vivid in your mind. Now, write it down as a small story in your note book or below.

Your Activating Event as a Recent, Memorable, Vivid Story

Now, we're going to identify the Critical A. I want you to either write down the aspect of your story that disturbs you the most, i.e. the most anxiety provoking aspect of the situation (if it's anxiety you are working on); or the most depressing aspect of the situation (if it's depression you are working on); or the most anger-provoking aspect, and so on. If you can't hit the nail on the head, write all the disturbing aspects of the situation as a list in your note book or overleaf.

The things about the situation that disturb you include:

Now that you have your list, identify the one thing that disturbs you the most – the Critical A – and then write it down below in the A column, not forgetting to include the resulting emotion at C.

A	C
My Activating Event is:	My emotion is:

Now, you're ready for the next part – formulating your beliefs. But first, you might want to take a break, because you've achieved a lot already. Take a break, imbibe a beverage, get some fresh air and then come back to this when you are ready. Unless you are ready now, in which case, read on.

Formulating Theo's Beliefs

By now, you are very familiar with the four thoughts that fuck you up, or the four unhealthy beliefs that can sit at B in the ABCDE model of psychological health. And so is Theo. I say 'can sit at B' because there is always a demand, but we don't know how many of the other three possible beliefs you hold in this situation. Not everyone awfulises, not everyone exhibits low frustration tolerance and not everyone puts themselves or others down. And, even if you do hold all three beliefs in the face of one particular demand, don't automatically assume that you will hold all three in the face of another demand attached to another problem. Always look for the demands, but the other three beliefs are assessed on a case-by-case basis.

So far, for Theo, we have:

A	C
Being judged by other people	Anxiety

Now, the demand is always the rigid version of the thing that disturbs you the most, it's the rigid version of the Critical A. It's the Critical A with a word such as 'must' or 'mustn't' or 'should' or 'shouldn't' in there.

For instance, if I have a tube train phobia and the thing that disturbs me the most is getting stuck in a tunnel, my demand will be 'I must not get stuck in a tunnel'. If I'm angry with my other half and the thing that disturbs me the most is that they don't respect me, then my demand is 'they must respect me'. Theo's problem is social anxiety, and the aspect of the problem that disturbs him the most is being judged by others, so his demand is 'I must not be judged by others', like so:

A		B	C
Being judged by other people	Dogmatic Demand	I must not be judged by other people	Anxiety

Now, we need to know if Theo is doing a 'drama', an 'I can't cope' or holding a 'put-down' in the face of this demand. We don't want to automatically assume that they are all there.

Remember that 'awful' is a rating of how bad it is that your demand is not met, and low frustration tolerance is a rating of your ability to deal with your demand not being met, while self-, other- or world-damning is a rating of yourself, others or 'things' if and when your demand is not met.

So, we asked Theo, when he was thinking of Beth's party and he was at his most disturbed, when he was really anxious about being judged by others: was it awful to him that other people could judge him – like, literally, the worst thing ever? If the answer is yes, it gets written down; if the answer is no, it does not get written down.

The important thing is to listen, not to your mind, but to your gut. Don't think about the answer, feel it. Your mind, given the situation you are in (reading this book in your case, in the therapy room in Theo's case), will be tempted to give the rational answer. But, we don't want the rational answer at this point, we want the irrational answer; we want the disturbance to talk. We don't want you to think, we want you to react. In this case, the answer was yes. If Theo went to Beth's party and other people judged him, it would be awful (literally, the worst thing he could imagine happening). So, now we have two beliefs:

A		B	C
Being judged by other people	Dogmatic Demand	I must not be judged by other people	Anxiety
	Dramas	It would be awful to be judged by other people	

Now, we must do the same thing with low frustration tolerance, when thinking about Beth's party and being judged by other people, when Theo was at his most anxious, would it be unbearable if he were judged? Again, we want to hear from Theo at his most anxious. We want the gut to answer, not the mind. Again, Theo's answer was yes. So, now we have three beliefs:

A		B	C
Being judged by other people	Dogmatic Demand	I must not be judged by other people	Anxiety
	Dramas	It would be awful to be judged by other people	
	I Can't Copes	I couldn't stand it if I was judged by other people	

Finally, we need to do the same thing with self-, other- or world-damning. Usually, with social anxiety, it's self-damning. When Theo was at his most anxious, was he putting himself down in any way? Don't forget that self-damning includes words such as useless, worthless, stupid, a failure, idiot, rubbish, no good, and so on. Theo said yes, and picked 'failure' and 'idiot' as his self-damning statements. So, now we have four beliefs and Theo's ABC looks like this:

A		B	C
Being judged by other people	Dogmatic Demand	I must not be judged by other people	Anxiety
	Dramas	It would be awful to be judged by other people	
	I Can't Copes	I couldn't stand it if I was judged by other people	
	Put-Downs	I'm a failure and an idiot if I am judged by other people	

So, this is what REBT says is going on whenever Theo thought about Beth's party. It triggered the belief 'I must not be judged by other people, it would be awful to be judged by other people, I couldn't stand it if I was judged by other people, and I'm a failure and an idiot if I am judged by other people'. It was this belief that triggered his anxiety, which meant that he forgot what he was doing sometimes, lost sleep in the days leading up to the event and, come the day, cancelled and did not attend.

To find out if we had hit the nail on the head, I simply asked Theo if this was an accurate representation of the problem. He replied with a resounding, 'Yes.'

Now, we need to look at the healthy equivalents to each belief. And to help remind you of those, here's another table:

Unhealthy beliefs	Healthy beliefs
I must have XYZ	I would prefer to have XYZ, but I don't have to have XYZ
It's awful not having XYZ	It will be bad if I don't have XYZ, but it won't be awful
I can't stand not having XYZ	I will find it difficult to deal with, but I know I can stand not having XYZ
I am a failure if I don't have XYZ	I'm not a failure, even if I don't have XYZ, I'm a worthwhile, fallible human being

Which means, Theo's healthy beliefs look like this:

A		B	C
Being judged by other people	Flexible Preference	I prefer not to be judged by other people, but there's no reason why I mustn't be	
	Perspective	It would be bad if I was judged by other people, but it would not be awful	
	I Can Cope	I would find it difficult to deal with if I was judged by other people, but I know I could stand it	
	Unconditional Acceptance	I'm not a failure or an idiot, even if I am judged by other people, I am a worthwhile, fallible human being	

Now, here is the million pound question. If Theo held these beliefs, if they were the default setting in his mind, how would he think, feel and act? Theo said that he would be worried about the possibility of being judged by other people but not anxious about it, and would feel more able to attend parties and social events with confidence. He added that, with this belief, he would definitely have been able to attend Beth's birthday party. And, just as importantly, if someone did judge him, while he may be upset by that judgement, he would not be destroyed by it.

Sounds like a winner, doesn't it? That is, a good belief system to work on and work towards. This goal is Theo's Effective rational outlook; the 'E' in the ABCDE model; it's the way he would think, and feel and act if he held those beliefs.

Formulating Your Unhealthy Beliefs

Now it's your turn. You have an A and you have a C. Now it's time to formulate your beliefs. Whatever you have identified at 'A' becomes a demand at B:

Not being in control $\rightarrow$ I must be in control

Not being respected $\rightarrow$ You must respect me

I didn't tell you $\rightarrow$ I should have told you

My life sucks $\rightarrow$ My life should not suck

Not getting into Valhalla $\rightarrow$ I must get into Valhalla

A		B	C
My Activating Event is:	Dogmatic Demand		My emotional Consequence is:

Once you have identified your demand, you can then move on to working out which of the other three beliefs you hold in the face of the demand. Don't forget, not everyone 'awfulises', not everyone exhibits 'low frustration tolerance' and not everyone puts themselves, others, or things down. Just ask yourself, when I am at my most disturbed, is it awful? When I am at my most disturbed, is it unbearable? When I am at my most disturbed, do I put others or myself down? Give the emotional answer here, go with your feelings, not with your head. If it feels awful, you hold that belief, if it feels unbearable, if only for a moment, you hold that belief and, if you feel like a failure, then you hold that belief.

If you don't think you're saying it, if you don't think you're thinking it, even when you are at your most disturbed, then there is no need to write it down.

A		B	C
My Activating Event is:	Dogmatic Demand		My emotional Consequence is:
	Dramas		
	I Can't Copes		
	Put-Downs		

Before you go any further, look at the beliefs you have written in your note book or above. These beliefs are what REBT says are triggering your disturbance (your unhealthy negative emotion). Do they sound like an accurate representation of the problem? If they do, you can move on to formulating healthy alternatives. If they do not, you may need to reflect on the above and go through the process again.

Formulating your healthy beliefs

Don't forget that the preference needs to 'negate' the demand. 'I must have XYZ' becomes 'I would prefer to have XYZ but I don't have to have it, or there's no law that says I must have it', while 'XYZ must not happen' becomes 'I would prefer, or I hope XYZ doesn't happen, but there is no reason why it shouldn't happen (or there is no law to say it must not happen)'.

The healthy alternative to awfulising still needs to take account of the 'badness' of the situation, and high frustration tolerance still needs to take account of the difficulty or the challenge of the situation, while self-, other- and world-acceptance need to take account of the worthwhile, fallible nature of all things.

A		B	C
My Activating Event is:	Flexible Preference		

	Perspective		
	I Can Cope		
	Unconditional Acceptance		

Now, for your million pound question: how would you think about your activating event if you held the above healthy beliefs? How would you feel and act? What other beneficial effects do you think you would notice? How would you feel if you didn't get the thing that you would prefer to have?

In short, do these beliefs sound like they would help you achieve your goal? Do they sound like a good belief system to work towards? They do? Awesome.

And there you have it, you now have an unhealthy set of beliefs that are the cause of your problem and you have a healthy set of beliefs that would change the way you think, feel and act and help you achieve your therapeutic and/or life goals.

Well done, you made it through the toughest chapter of the book. Now, let's have a look at the Stuff to Do and then you're more or less done for the week.

Stuff to Do for Week Two

- Learn your beliefs, both the unhealthy and the healthy. Memorise them so well that, if someone were to ask you what they were, you could repeat them word for word, without looking at what you have written.

Before you start the Week Three chapter, just answer the following reflective questions:

Reflective Questions

- What is this chapter about?
- Can you relate the beliefs that you have identified to any other areas of your life?
- Have you had any insights, or 'light bulb' moments as a result of reading through this chapter, learning your beliefs and reflecting on what other areas they may relate to over this past week?

Week Three

Questioning the Validity of Your Thoughts

Intellectual growth should commence at birth and cease only at death.

Albert Einstein

When your unhealthy beliefs hold sway, rationality runs away. It plays a really hard game of hide and seek. Later on, when you've calmed down, that rationality will have slipped back in unnoticed, and you'll be wondering why the hell you made such a big deal of something that wasn't such a big deal in the first place. This is why challenging your beliefs is important. REBT can give you the tools to be rational in the moments when you are not. It can teach you to think before you react.

And so, now that you have identified your unhealthy beliefs and developed healthy alternatives, it's time to move on to the 'D' in the ABCDE model of psychological health.

Here, 'D' stands for disputing, which is just a posh word for challenging. D is the process of challenging your beliefs over and over again, and in doing so, weakening your conviction in your unhealthy beliefs and strengthening your conviction in your healthy beliefs. There are various exercises in that process that, little by little, help effect a shift in the way you think, feel and act.

You've already been introduced to the first disputing exercise, known as 'disputing arguments' or 'disputation' – it was a thread that ran through Parts One and Two of this book as you were introduced to all four unhealthy beliefs and all four healthy beliefs. But, we're going to go through it here again, just for good measure. That may seem a little repetitive, but it's important for two very good reasons.

Firstly, disputing is the foundation stone of everything we do in challenging your beliefs, without it in place, you'll be on very dodgy ground (emotionally, at least) going forwards. Secondly, repetition is key; it's how we learn. It's how things sink in and stay sunk in for good, and has been ever since we were little.

Let's say I asked you, 'What's three multiplied by three?' or, 'What are six sixes?' You may be a little surprised that I've just randomly chucked a maths question or two into a self-help therapy book, but I'm hoping that you answered '9' and '36' respectively, pretty quickly and, more importantly, without using a calculator, your fingers or a pencil. Because '9' and '36' are ingrained in your mind as the de facto answers to those two particular questions. There's no need to question them, or check them, because you know them. But, how did they get there?

Well, they got there through sheer repetition. Probably in a similar fashion to myself, at school as a little kid, standing up with everyone else in the class and reciting my times tables over and over again, until they become indelibly etched upon my memory.

And that's what we need to do, not only with 'disputation' arguments, but all the exercises that follow it. In order to effect a shift, in order to change your beliefs and in order to gain control of your unhealthy negative emotion, repetition is key.

A Quick Reintroduction to Disputing

If you remember, disputing involved the use of three questions, or three challenges. Those questions are:

1. Is this belief true?
2. Does this belief make sense?
3. Does this belief help me?

These questions are applied to each one of your unhealthy beliefs, one by one; and to each one of your healthy beliefs, again one by one. Don't forget that these questions are used everywhere: maths, science, philosophy, and more. They are excellent for challenging, well, pretty much anything – to see what holds up and what falls down, be it a piece of scientific research, a philosophical musing or a political point of view. And this is exactly what we need to do to your beliefs.

'Is it true?' is the science question, or the court of law question, as it wants proof; it is asking for evidence to support your statement. 'Does it make sense?' is the logical, or common sense question; 'just because you think ABC', it asks, 'does it logically follow that XYZ'? Finally, 'does it help me?' is the most obvious question. You have a goal. You are simply asking if that particular belief helps you to achieve that goal or not.

Disputing is an excellent skill to use both philosophically and therapeutically. When was the last time you challenged the validity of your thoughts? Or challenged their logic and usefulness, either directly to yourself or in the results that they bring? How many thoughts do you think you're operating according to right now that manage to be both invalid and illogical, as well as unhelpful? What would it mean to you if you dropped those thoughts? What would you get if you replaced them with thoughts that were not only valid and logical, but that also helped you or brought you the results that you wanted?

Let's remind ourselves of the beliefs we can hold:

Dogmatic Demands: Demands are never true. If they were, you would get them 100 per cent of the time, you would have always got them, and you could guarantee you always would. Demands don't make sense. Just because you would like something to happen, it does not logically follow that it has to happen. Demands don't help you; they disturb you, they fuck you up.

Dramas: Awfulising thoughts are not true, because you can always think of something worse. Just because something is bad, it does not logically follow that it is awful. Saying it is awful does not help you, it makes a situation worse than it actually is and it turns you into a bit of a drama queen.

I Can't Copes: Believing that you can't cope or stand something is not true. If you truly couldn't stand something, it would kill you. It doesn't make any sense to believe you can't stand something, just because you find it difficult to deal with. It does not help you to believe this. It weakens you, it disempowers you and it makes it more likely that other unhealthy coping strategies will creep in.

Pejorative Put-Downs: It's not true to say you are useless, stupid, or an idiot. Everything you have ever got right, everything you have ever achieved is positive proof that you are not. This is equally true of others. It's the same with 'world' conditions too. Just because you, or someone else, has failed at something, it does not logically follow that you or they are a complete failure. The world can't be totally horrible, because it has nice things in it. And putting people and situations down does not help you.

So, unhealthy beliefs are not true, do not make sense and do not help you. It's another matter entirely for your healthy beliefs:

Flexible Preferences: Preferences are always true. If you say you would prefer to have something, then it is true for you. But, if you haven't got it, then believing 'there is no reason why you must have it' or 'there is no law to say you must have it ' simply acknowledges that fact. Preferences also make sense. It's perfectly logical to accept that you don't always get what you want, even though you want it very much. Preferences also help you, in that they promote good mental health.

Perspectives: When you believe something is bad, but not awful, you can prove it to be true. If you don't like something, then it's bad. But, as you can always think of worse things that can happen (or have happened), then you can prove it's not awful. Saying something is bad, or that you don't like it is sensible. Saying that the bad thing is not an awful thing is equally sensible. Believing something is bad but not awful will always help you keep a sense of perspective.

I Can Copes: Believing that something is difficult to deal with but you know that you can cope with it is true. Your emotions, the way you react, and even a complete breakdown is evidence that you might find the situation difficult, but the fact that you are alive to tell the tale proves that you can cope with it. Admitting that you find something difficult or challenging is rational, but concluding that you know you can deal with this difficult, challenging thing is equally rational. Believing this also helps you; it empowers you, it helps you to cope with adversity.

Unconditional Acceptance: You can prove you are not a failure because your successes are evidence. You can prove you are not stupid because the things at which you are good are proof; plus you can prove the same for other people. The world is not a totally horrible place because it has positive things in it, and your job is not complete crap because there will be things about your job that you like. You can prove you are fallible, because you make mistakes. Everybody does, therefore everybody is fallible. You can even prove your job to be fallible. It's not perfect, is it? And, when it comes to human beings, we are all equal, we all have worth, and we are all worthwhile. Therefore the belief

'I am not a failure, I am a worthwhile, fallible human being' is true. Now, while it's rational to rate individual aspects of the self and others (as in, I am good at this, but not good at that), it is also rational to accept one's self and others as worthwhile, fallible human beings. One statement logically flows from the other. If you base your confidence not on your 'stuff', but on your innate worth as a human being, good and bad, right and wrong, warts and all, you'll feel much more confident.

Your healthy beliefs are true, do make sense and do help you. They keep you calm and rational.

So, that's disputing in a nutshell (and repeated, but with just cause). It is a very rational, objective exercise, designed to help you think intellectually about the problem, rather than react emotionally to it.

When people go through the disputing exercise, especially when with me in the therapy room, they often claim that I'm just pointing out the bleeding obvious.[1] It's an accusation to which I happily agree. I am indeed pointing out the bleeding obvious. As I mentioned earlier, when your unhealthy beliefs kick in, rationality leaves the building. And, when it does that, you are most definitely not pointing out the bleeding obvious to yourself. You'll have either lost the plot, or the red-mist will have descended or it will be all forest and no trees for you.

---

[1] A sarcastic English euphemism that means something is so evident that it goes without saying. Until a few decades ago, 'bloody' was considered a very naughty word indeed.

Disputing is a very clear-cut technique that allows you to be rational and objective, even if your emotions are trying to tell you something else.[2]

Theo's Disputing Arguments

First, we are going to apply disputing arguments to each one of Theo's unhealthy beliefs about being judged by other people, and then to each one of his healthy beliefs about being judged by other people. And then, you are going to apply them to the beliefs you identified in the previous chapter.

When Theo pointed out the bleeding obvious to himself, it looked a lot like this:

I must not be judged by other people

1. This belief is not true, because I have been judged by other people in the past and I will probably be judged by other people again in the future.
2. Just because I prefer not to be judged, it does not logically follow that I must not be judged. One is rational (I prefer not to be judged) and the other is irrational (I must not be judged) so one does not logically flow from the other.

---

[2] Feelings are not facts, not always, and not when you hold unhealthy beliefs. Just because something feels awful, it doesn't mean it is awful. When you hold healthy beliefs, you can call your feelings 'intuition' and trust them more.

3. This belief does not help me; it makes me anxious, too
    anxious to go to parties and social events. This also
    means I am more likely to be judged negatively by
    others. My friends judge me for not going and other
    people judge me as nervous and awkward if and
    when they do meet me.

It's awful when other people judge me

1. This is not true. It is not 100 per cent bad, because
    I can think of worse things that could happen than
    being judged.
2. It doesn't make sense to say judgement is awful, just
    because I don't like it. They're two different things.
    One is rational (I don't like being judged); the other
    is irrational (therefore it is awful being judged). One
    does not logically follow from the other.
3. It doesn't help me to say this. Instead, it blows
    everything out of proportion and makes it worse than
    it actually is. I don't just react, I overreact; and that's
    not good.

I can't stand it when other people judge me

1. This belief is not true. I have been judged before and I
    have survived, it didn't kill me. I am the proof that this
    statement is not true.
2. I don't like judgement. I mean, who would? Maybe
    I find it a little harder to deal with than others but it
    doesn't mean I can't stand it. 'I find it difficult' is one
    thing, 'I can't stand it' is another, completely different
    thing. One does not logically flow from the other.

3. The belief does not help me but, because I believe it, I avoid socialising as much as possible. Avoidance has become my way of coping.

I am a failure and an idiot if I am judged by other people

1. This belief is not true. I have qualifications, I hold down a job, I have hobbies and interests, I have family and friends that like me for who I am, therefore it is not true to say these things.

2. It doesn't make sense to believe this. Okay, so socialising is not my strong point. I'm not very good at it and, as a result, probably do get judged negatively about it, but it's my behaviour they are judging. Maybe my behaviour is stupid, but it does not logically follow that I am stupid because of it. They are two different things and one does not logically flow from the other.

3. This belief does not help me. In fact, it saps my confidence and, if I do actually socialise, it increases the likelihood that I will be judged negatively. It makes me actively dislike myself.

I would prefer it if other people didn't judge me, but there's no reason why they mustn't

1. It's true that I would prefer not to be judged. Actually, it's probably true for everybody, but it's so true for me that I've turned it into a bit of a problem. But, people can judge me, have judged me and probably will judge me in the future so, given that,

it is equally true that there's no reason why they mustn't do that.

2. Saying I prefer not to be judged is rational. Accepting that people can and do judge, even if I don't want them to, is equally rational. One statement logically follows from the other.

3. This belief would help me to accept the possibility of judgement which, in turn, would help keep me calmer about the whole thing. It would allow me to walk into a room without panicking.

It would be bad if other people judged me, but it wouldn't be awful

1. This belief is true. I won't like it if other people judge me (therefore it is bad), but I'm not ill, homeless, destitute or friendless, so I can think of worse (therefore it is not awful).

2. Saying I don't like it is rational, accepting that it is not awful is equally rational; one statement logically flows from the other.

3. This belief would help me; it would give me a sense of perspective. I would see 'judgement' for what it is, rather than turning it into something it isn't.

I would find it difficult to deal with if other people judged me, but I know I could stand it

1. This statement is entirely true. I do find it difficult to deal with (my anxiety is proof of that), but I know I can stand it because I won't die.

2. Saying I find it difficult is rational, saying that I can stand the difficulty of negative judgement is also rational. One logically flows from the other.

3. This belief would help me; it would help me to deal with negative judgement, if there even was any. More importantly, it would help me to socialise.

I am not a failure, or an idiot, even if other people judge me; I am a worthwhile, fallible human being

1. This belief is totally true: I have successes and achievements, things I am good at, so I cannot be a failure; I also have things I am not good at, things I am rubbish at, I've made mistakes and failed at things, so I am fallible; I am also worthwhile, we all are.
2. Acknowledging my failings is rational; accepting myself as a worthwhile, fallible human being in the face of my flaws is equally rational. One statement logically follows from the other.
3. This belief would help me, it would give me confidence in myself. I would be comfortable with who I am and I would be able to socialise with others, even if socialising is not my strong point.

So, there you have it. Theo's unhealthy beliefs are not true, do not make sense and do not help him achieve his goal; while his healthy beliefs are true, do make sense and would help him achieve his goal.

Now, it's your turn. I want you to take what you have learnt from this chapter (and from all the information on disputing in Parts One and Two of this book) and apply it to your specific beliefs. You can copy what you have read above, more or less word for word if you want, but I would prefer it if you used what you learnt in Parts One and Two as well as the above, and then used all of it as a springboard to dispute your beliefs in your own way, using your own language and style.

And (if you don't like writing things down) feel free to record yourself disputing your beliefs.[3]

My Dogmatic Demand is . . .

_____

_____

1. It is not true, here's why . . .

_____

_____

_____

2. It does not make sense, here's why . . .

_____

_____

_____

---

[3] Quite a lot of people record their 'stuff to do' using the voice memo function on their smartphones and bring them into their next session with me.

3. It does not help me, here's why . . .

_____

_____

_____

My Doing a Drama belief is . . .

_____

_____

1. It is not true, here's why . . .

_____

_____

_____

2. It does not make sense, here's why . . .

_____

_____

_____

3. It does not help me, here's why . . .

_____

_____

_____

My I Can't Cope belief is . . .

_____

_____

1. It is not true, here's why . . .

_____

_____

_____

2. It does not make sense, here's why . . .

_____

_____

_____

3. It does not help me, here's why . . .

_____

_____

_____

My Pejorative Put-Down belief is . . .

_____

_____

1. It is not true, here's why . . .

_____

_____

_____

2. It does not make sense, here's why . . .

_____

_____

_____

3. It does not help me, here's why . . .

_____

_____

_____

My Flexible Preference belief is . . .

_____

_____

1. It is true, here's why . . .

_____

_____

2. It does make sense, here's why . . .

_____

_____

_____

3. It does help me, here's why . . .

_____

_____

_____

My Possessing Perspective belief is . . .

_____

_____

1. It is true, here's why . . .

_____

_____

_____

2. It does make sense, here's why . . .

_____

_____

_____

3. It does help me, here's why . . .

_____

_____

_____

My I Can Cope belief is . . .

_____

_____

1. It is true, here's why . . .

_____

_____

_____

2. It does make sense, here's why . . .

_____

_____

_____

3. It does help me, here's why . . .

_____

_____

_____

My Unconditional Acceptance belief is . . .

_____

_____

1. It is true, here's why . . .

_____

_____

_____

2. It does make sense, here's why . . .

_____

_____

_____

3. It does help me, here's why . . .

_____

_____

_____

Stuff to Do for Week Three

- Read through your disputing arguments several times over the week, reflect on them and try to apply them to your specific problem. (Don't worry if they don't have an effect, that is not the point at this time, the aim is to get into the habit of thinking rationally and objectively.)
- Try and apply what you have learnt here to other situations and scenarios in your daily life as you encounter them. So, if you notice yourself saying or thinking a demand, or that something is awful, or unbearable, or you call yourself or someone else an idiot, take a step back and challenge the belief.

Before you start the Week Four chapter next week, answer the following reflective questions:

Reflective Questions

- What is this chapter about and how have you applied it?
- Can you relate 'disputing your beliefs' to any other areas of your life? Have you tried to do so and, if so, to what effect?
- Have you had any insights or 'light bulb' moments as a result of reading through this chapter, disputing your beliefs and reflecting on what other areas they may relate to over the past week?

Week Four
What you Say is What you Get

If you wish to persuade me, you must think my thoughts, feel my feelings, and speak my words.

Cicero

So, by now, if you have followed the steps in this part of the book, you will have identified a problem and formulated the unhealthy beliefs that are the cause of your emotional and behavioural reactions to that problem, and formulated the healthy alternatives that could bring about a much more rational and beneficial outcome for all concerned. Said unhealthy beliefs will definitely contain a demand, and also at least one of the following derivative beliefs, if not more: an awfulising belief, a low frustration tolerance belief and a self-, other- or world-damning belief. And the healthy beliefs will contain the rational equivalents to each one.

Hopefully, you will also have disputed those beliefs. But, I bet you're still disturbed, right? You are still thinking, feeling and acting the same way that you always did.

Sure, you may have noticed a shift in the way you deal with some things. Other things. But, they're the lesser things, the not-so-disturbing things. When it comes to the big things, the things you really are disturbing yourself about and really do want to get under your control, you're still reacting the same way. It's a bummer, I know, but, at this stage, it's also totally appropriate to where you are.

Many years ago I had a client who came to me with a tube train phobia. When we were disputing his beliefs, he had an epiphany, especially when it came to his dramas and I can't copes.

The epiphany was obvious by his expression, so I asked him what he was thinking. 'I've just massively understood my whole life,' he said. 'I've realised I've always been stressed because if anything goes even a tiny bit wrong, I will catastrophise it and I'm always saying, "I can't stand this, and I can't stand that." I was stressed at college and university and I'm stressed at work all the time, and for what? I'm not doing that anymore.'

And he didn't; he made good on his word. In fact, he was so calm and relaxed over the following week, both personally and professionally, that his friends, family and colleagues kept joking and saying, 'Who are you and what have you done with Simon?'

So relaxed was his week that he decided to surprise me. It was raining and he opted to travel to his next appointment by tube train, despite this not having been set as homework yet. He was right about one thing though. I was surprised because, when I opened my door, I opened it to a soaking wet, hyperventilating mess, gibbering incoherently and not understanding why he had just had a panic attack.

Although he only worked a short journey away from me, five stops at most, everything that could go wrong had gone wrong. Everything that could possibly trigger his unhealthy beliefs had happened.

For a start there had been torrential rain. Some tube stations had flooded and closed down. The adverse weather had caused signal failures on several lines, so that every station was full, the trains were slow and packed to the roof with hot, angry, wet people.

There Simon sat, in his seat on his train, trying not to have a panic attack, reciting his beliefs over and over again, both unhealthy and healthy, and disputing them as loudly as possible in his head, and even muttering them under his breath. And yet, he could feel his panic rising. To the point where it overwhelmed him, to the point where he freaked out and forced his way off the train, screaming 'Let me out, let me out, let me out!'

And then he disturbed himself even more because he had tried to use REBT and failed miserably. The only conclusions in his mind at that point were either that therapy didn't work, or that he was no good at it.

As I have mentioned before, REBT is a great guide for everyday living, which is why Simon had applied it so successfully to his everyday life. Sometimes, just using the language is enough to course correct a few unhealthy, but habitual reactions, to things. However, using it as an effective form of psychotherapy in the face of a specific disturbance, as opposed to a philosophy for life in general, requires more effort. Disputing your day-to-day thoughts is one thing; disputing your deeply held, disturbance-causing beliefs is another.

Simon had used disputing to good effect in his day-to-day-life, but it didn't help yet when it came to the things he was truly irrational about.

As the old adage goes, don't try to run before you can walk. Also, if you do have a tube train phobia, don't get on a tube train until you've agreed it as a homework assignment with your therapist.

The problem is this: rationally, logically and objectively, you know your unhealthy beliefs are not true, do not make sense and do not help you; and yet, you go there with a practised ease. They are still your default setting. They just come automatically to you, they are still your natural way of thinking.

Your healthy beliefs, on the other hand – well, sure, you know they are true, you know they do make sense and you know they could help you, but they don't feel right, you don't believe them and you are not really convinced by them. They are not your natural way of thinking. Not yet.

What we have developed so far throughout this book is an intellectual understanding of the problem and of the beliefs behind it. But, in order to effect a shift in the way you think, feel and act, we also have to develop what we call emotional understanding.

Simply put, intellectual understanding is *knowing* what to do, while emotional understanding is *believing* that you can do it. Intellectual understanding always needs to be worked on first. It is the foundation stone on which everything else is based. Without it, your unhealthy negative emotions will hold sway. Once we have that rational foundation in place, we can start chipping away at the emotional conviction that has you favouring your unhealthy beliefs.

It's Not Only What You Say, It's Also How You Say It

Which is where the 'persuasive arguments technique' comes in. With this, you will be developing really meaningful, emotive and complex arguments that undermine these unhealthy beliefs. Arguments that help you to let go of them and stop using them. At the same time, you'll be building equally meaningful, emotive and complex arguments that help you to reinforce your healthy beliefs. The technique helps you to become more convinced by the healthy technique than you currently are, and be more inclined to put them into practice, despite them not yet being your natural way of thinking.

This needs to be done in a structured and sustained way. We still look at your unhealthy beliefs, one by one, and still look at your healthy beliefs, one by one, and we still attack them with questions, but, this time, the questions are more personal.

Before you start this exercise, I will show you examples of persuasive arguments, but don't just copy and paste what I've written, or use them as a springboard for your arguments. In order to be truly 'persuasive', these arguments need to come from you. For two main reasons, they really do need to be personal. So, you're going to need to dig deep.

The first reason they need to come from you is because, essentially, all persuasion is self-persuasion.[1]

Advertising does not persuade very many people of anything. Advertisers spend millions on advertising – to create brand awareness, to get you to buy into their product and

---

[1] According to some sociologists it is, as least.

to make money. But adverts do not persuade you to buy into anything. You do. You look at the advert and you decide whether you want to buy or not. You are the one that goes, 'Hmm, yes, I would like to try that.' Equally, you could look at that advert, take it all in, appreciate it even, and yet conclude, 'No, thanks.' And that would be it.

Let's say you and I meet socially at a party. And we get talking. And the conversation turns towards one of the big topics: politics, religion and so on. You have one point of view and I have the diametrically opposed point of view. We've had a couple of drinks and so the conversation is animated, not in a nasty way, but in a passionate way, where the alcohol may have loosened our tongues just a tad. By the end of the conversation I have convinced you of my point of view. Except, I didn't convince you, I did not persuade you. You did all that yourself. You are the one that weighed everything up in your mind and decided to change your mind. It doesn't matter how passionate I was, or how well I argued my case, you actually listened to your own internal monologue and then decided to side with me. If you had persuaded yourself otherwise, there would be nothing I could do about it.

Talking of drinks. Not so long ago, a friend of mine was given a bottle of salted caramel vodka as a birthday present. And, why not? She was a fan of pretty much anything that contained the words 'salted' and 'caramel' in them. And she liked vodka. She was also partial to the occasional espresso martini, which contains a shot of espresso coffee, a shot of coffee liqueur and, you guessed it, a shot of vodka.

'I wonder if there's a salted caramel vodka espresso martini?' she mused. And then promptly Googled it. A recipe for such a cocktail did exist. Many such recipes in fact. And, for a full, deep, rich and satisfying espresso martini experience, practically all the recipes recommend a thick, strong shot of espresso from a coffee machine instead of the more watered-down, not-so-rich-and-satisfying instant version. Which got her thinking.

'I do like coffee,' she thought. 'And buying it from a coffee shop is expensive, and not very environmentally friendly because they're always "to go". My cups would be for keeps if I made it at home. And it would be nice to have salted caramel espresso martini nights with friends. And, as I've said, I drink coffee. Often. So, a coffee machine would be a good thing to have. Almost essential, really, when you think about it.'

And so, she bought a £200 premium espresso coffee machine. All because someone bought her a bottle of salted caramel vodka. That's the power of self-persuasion. It's an aspect of social influence theory, which says that you are taking an active role in persuading yourself to change your behaviour. If I try to persuade you, it is direct. And the motivation to change is external, from me to you. If you persuade yourself, it is indirect and internal. I'm encouraging you to change, for sure, so I'm an influence, but the motivation comes from within. Self-persuasion is considered the deeper and more long-lasting of the two.

The other reason these arguments need to come from you is that, in order to be persuasive, they need to be personal. This means they can only come from you. They have to contain examples and anecdotes drawn from your personal experience.

Imagine that I am running a social anxiety group attended by 10 people, including Theo. Social anxiety is usually, but not exclusively, a fear of negative judgement, which is the basis of Theo's anxiety. Let's say all 10 people have exactly the same beliefs about that negative judgement, such as 'I must not be judged, it would be awful to be judged, I couldn't stand it if I was judged and, if I am judged, it's because I am useless, inept and rubbish'.

Now, when we dispute those beliefs, all ten people would give me the same answers. Irrespective of their differing ages, genders and cultural backgrounds, their answers would all be 'no, no, no' for the unhealthy beliefs and 'yes, yes, yes' for the healthy beliefs. However, when it comes to developing persuasive arguments, each person would give different answers and discuss different examples.

This is because each one of those 10 people, despite sharing the same unhealthy anxiety provoking beliefs, have led very different lives and have been affected by those beliefs at different points, at different times, with different outcomes. In short, their personal stories would be different. So you're going to have to dig deep and get personal.

Good questions to ask when formulating your persuasive arguments are:

- What do I get when I hold this belief?
- How do I think, feel and act when I hold this belief?
- What does this belief make me do?
- What does this belief prevent me from doing?
- Who else does this belief affect?
- What outcomes do I get with this belief, and do I like those outcomes?

Before we look at what a persuasive argument is, let me explain what it is not.

This is not a persuasive argument:

Belief: 'Other people must not get in my way'
'I get angry with people that get in my way'

It's true, in that I do get angry with the people that get in my way; that certainly hits the nail on the head. But, this sentence doesn't tell me anything about how these beliefs have been affecting my life. To be persuasive, it needs to be drawn from my personal experience, so I need to dredge up examples from the past. So will you, when you formulate yours. Think of them as a potted history of you, drawn through the filter of your unhealthy and healthy beliefs.

With that in mind, here are some persuasive arguments that tell me more about what is going on.

Other people must not get in my way

1. With this belief I make myself angry before I've even gone anywhere. I anticipate the crowds and people in advance. If friends invite me anywhere, my first thought is, 'Oh no.'
2. With this belief, god forbid anyone who actually does get in my way, I'm really quite rude. And that's the polite end of the spectrum.
3. Because of this belief I don't want to go anywhere, I limit myself. I don't like going to concerts or festivals, or even bars and clubs. Not because those things are not my cup of tea, because they are, but because I know they will be full of people getting in my way. I said no to a night out last week because of this.

4. I go from zero to angry in a few minutes with this belief, in any crowded space, and angry me mutters under his breath, swears, growls, tells people off and even shoves them out of the way. Just like I did at Oxford Street tube station on Saturday.

I would prefer it if other people did not get in my way, but there is no reason why they mustn't

1. With this belief I would be much calmer in any and all crowded situations, which is better for me, better for them and better for the people that I am with. I'd be more relaxed and people would relax more with me.
2. With this belief my social life would improve, I would be able to go to crowded bars, clubs and concerts. Instead of storming off (which is what I did the last time someone managed to persuade me to go clubbing), I would be able to stay the course and enjoy my evening.
3. Travelling at rush hour with this belief would be a very different experience. Instead of gearing myself up for it, I wouldn't even think about it and I'd just take it in my stride when I have to.
4. I would be able to trust myself more in crowded situations, as I know I wouldn't be kicking off at anyone any time soon.

I hope you can see that my arguments are complex, emotive and contain a few anecdotes drawn from my personal experience.

As with disputing, you develop persuasive arguments for each and every unhealthy and healthy belief you have identified. You are arguing against your unhealthy beliefs and what they are getting you, but arguing for your healthy beliefs and what they could get you.

Try to develop as many arguments as possible for each belief. The more arguments you can develop with the more personal detail – the more you are persuading yourself. By the end of this exercise, and by putting it into practice, you should notice a shift in the way you think, feel and act, to some degree or another.

In essence you are creating two pictures in your mind: one of a life lived according to your currently held unhealthy beliefs (which is not going to be very pleasant, and will be awash with dysfunctional feelings, behaviours and outcomes); and one of a life that could be yours if you lived it according to your healthy beliefs (which will look far more pleasant, and be replete with functional feelings, behaviours and outcomes). More importantly still, you will realise that this picture is neither utopian, nor unobtainable.

When Theo developed his persuasive arguments, they looked like this:

What do I get when I tell myself 'I must not be judged'?

1. With this belief, I pull out of practically every party and social event I have ever been invited to. I make excuses and I lie, just like I did with Beth's party. I wanted to go but, in the end, I couldn't. I bailed on her.
2. Because of this belief my university experience was quite lonely and miserable. My friendships were cursory and faded soon after. I envy my friend who went to university at the same time as me and forged several long-lasting friendships.

3. It affects me in my current job, it's affected me in all the jobs I've had. People from work socialise and I don't socialise with them. I feel it has created distance with my colleagues. It happened last Friday; almost everyone went out for a drink after work and I did not join them.

4. This belief has affected my friendship with Beth. She is so pissed off with me at the moment.

What do I get when I tell myself 'it is awful when other people judge me'?

1. With this belief I am blowing everything out of proportion; I've decided that everyone in the room already has an opinion about me, which is a bit much.

2. Not only that but I have decided that everyone will have a negative opinion of me; it does not allow for positive opinions, or no opinions at all.

3. This belief gives me a sense of humour bypass. I can be quite funny really, but not when I believe this and I'm in a group situation. Then I go quiet, I become bland and monotone.

What do I get when I tell myself 'I can't stand being judged by other people'?

1. Right there, with this belief, this is why I bail. This is why I don't go to things. This is why I say no. Because I believe I can't stand it; I avoid normal, human social interaction.

2. Because of this belief, I monitor myself when I do socialise (which is rare). I second guess myself, so I don't say or do anything that could be judged. This makes me

appear inauthentic which, in turn, makes it more likely I will be judged. I've actually had people tell me they find it hard to get to know me or don't know who I am.

3. Because of this belief, if people do actually judge me negatively or I hear that they have, I fall to pieces. I've had panic attacks before. At university I would walk the other way or hide if I saw this one particular guy who I knew didn't like me.

I'm a failure and an idiot if I am judged by other people

1. This belief makes me berate myself, I beat myself up for my perceived inadequacies and my social ineptitude which, in turn, makes me even more awkward in social situations.

2. On several occasions, I've actually agreed with people who have put me down. I've done that my whole life, through school, through university and at work.

3. I'm judging myself with this belief. Before I've given anyone else the chance to judge me either positively or negatively, I've judged myself. It saps my confidence and makes me insecure. I am insecure with my girlfriend and constantly wonder what she even sees in me.

I would prefer not to be judged by others but there is no reason why I mustn't

1. This belief would take the pressure off me. I would accept reality – that people judge other people, that it goes on all the time. In fact, it's normal. When I normalise it, I don't have to hide away from it.

2. My whole life would have been completely different with this belief, all of it – childhood, school, university, work, you name it. It would have produced a calmer, happier me then, and it would do the same, starting now, if I believed it.

3. With this belief I would say 'yes' to the things I wanted to attend and 'no' to the things I didn't want to attend. More importantly, I wouldn't be saying no because I was scared, I would be saying no because I genuinely didn't want to go, or had other plans. I would definitely have gone to Beth's party with this belief.

It's bad when other people judge me, but it is not awful

1. This puts things into perspective. With this belief I realise that not everyone is out to get me, that some people will like me, some people won't and some people will even be indifferent. That's not so bad now, is it?

2. With this belief, I won't spend ages fretting or second-guessing what other people think, my mind will be free, free to keep calm, free to concentrate on other things, free to just relax and enjoy myself.

3. I will be able to attend social events with this belief as I won't be worried about making a good impression. I won't be clamming up, I won't be sick with dread; I will be relaxed and it will allow people to meet the real me who, I am told, is quite nice really.

I will find it difficult to deal with other people judging me, but I know I can stand it

1. This belief gives me strength and it gives me confidence. I can walk into a room, a bar or a club, anywhere really, with my head held high. I will be able to make eye contact with people. I've always wanted to be able to do that properly.

2. This belief allows me to be me, someone who finds socialising difficult, so I know I'm not going to be the most confident person in the room but, more importantly, I will be in the room.

3. My friendships will improve. People won't feel let down by me because I won't be letting them down. Friends will be happy for me, because they don't like me being the other way either. It's the same with my family. In fact, my social life will improve because people will learn that they can invite me to stuff and can trust that I will turn up.

I am not a failure or an idiot, even if other people judge me; I am a worthwhile, fallible human being

1. With this belief, I will believe in myself. Other people will be free to make up their own minds, but their opinions will be based on the real me, not the anxious, riddled-with-doubt me.

2. There will be no more sitting at home on my own feeling like a loser with this belief; my weekends

are going to look very different now. In fact, if I am sitting at home on my own at all, it will be because I want to.

3. I will feel free with this belief. Free from self-doubt and free to be the real me. I may even be able to look forward to social events with excitement instead of dread. The future is full of possibilities. There's a birthday party coming up in a month. I could actually attend. With this belief, I know I could.

Over to You

Now, it's your turn to formulate persuasive arguments that look at what your unhealthy beliefs have been getting you and what your healthy beliefs could get you. Try to make the arguments as complex, emotive and personal as possible. Try to include real-world examples from your life, from your history, in relation to the problem you are working on. Remember, good questions to ask yourself to help you formulate your arguments are:

- What do I get when I hold this belief?
- How do I think, feel and act when I hold this belief?
- What does this belief make me do?
- What does it prevent me from doing?
- How does it affect me?
- How does it affect other people?
- What outcomes do I get with this belief and do I like those outcomes?

Try to develop as many arguments for your belief as possible; the more arguments you can develop the more you are persuading yourself. However, we don't want you to go on and on for the sake of it. The purpose of this exercise is not to come up with arguments for the sake of coming up with arguments, but to effect a shift in the way you think, feel and act in relation to the problem you are working on.

Kindle and tablet people, and all those who prefer not to write in their books it's back to the pad and the pen for you; otherwise, write here:

My Dogmatic Demand belief is ...

_____

_____

What it gets me is ...

_____

_____

_____

_____

_____

My Doing a Drama belief is ...

_____

_____

What it gets me is ...

_____

_____

_____

_____

_____

My I Can't Cope belief is ...

_____

_____

What it gets me is ...

_____

_____

_____

_____

My Pejorative Put-Down belief is ...

_____

_____

What it gets me is ...

_____

_____
_____
_____
_____

My Flexible Preference belief is ...

_____
_____

What it gets me is ...

_____
_____
_____
_____

My Possessing Perspective belief is ...

_____
_____

What it gets me is ...

_____
_____
_____

_____

_____

My I Can Cope belief is ...

_____

_____

What it gets me is ...

_____

_____

_____

_____

_____

My Unconditional Acceptance belief is ...

_____

_____

What it gets me is ...

_____

_____

_____

_____

_____

Stuff to Do for Week Four

- Read through your persuasive arguments several times over the coming week, reflect on them and try to apply them to your specific problem. Make a note of any and all effects you notice as a result of using these arguments.
- Note down your success and your doubts in this respect (i.e. notice what improvement you have made, but also identify any blocks to moving forwards that appear). And don't beat yourself up if things don't go as well as you would like. There are no failures, only opportunities to learn.

Before you start the chapter on Week Five, just answer the following reflective questions:

Reflective Questions

- What is this chapter about and how have you applied that knowledge?
- Can you relate 'persuasive arguments' to any other areas of your life? Have you tried to do so and, if so, to what effect?
- Have you noticed an emotional shift and, if so, to what degree? What changes in your mood and/or behaviour have you noticed?

Week Five
Repeat, Repeat, Repeat

We are what we repeatedly do. Excellence, then, is not an act, but a habit.

Will Durant

You now have two tools in your REBT toolkit that help you to challenge your unhealthy beliefs and reinforce your healthy beliefs, namely disputing and persuasive arguments. How much that has helped you thus far, I cannot say, mainly because everybody is different. Some of you may have attempted to face your challenges and some not, some of you may already be feeling very different about the problem you are working on and some of you may only feel slightly different. There's a good reason for that. It all depends on how much you believe in your healthy beliefs at this point. It hinges on how much conviction you hold in them overall.

So, here is an important question: if you could rate your conviction in your healthy beliefs as a percentage right now, what would that percentage be? I'm not talking about how much you understand them (intellectually, in your head); I mean how much do you believe in them, right now (emotionally, in your heart)? If you were to face the thing that disturbs you, right here and right now, then as a percentage, how much would you be convinced by your healthy beliefs? Whatever that percentage is, write it down:

My conviction in my healthy beliefs is: %

What did you put? Was it 10 per cent, or 20 per cent? Was it higher? Was it more like 50 per cent, or higher still, say, something like 70 per cent? More importantly, what does that figure tell us? Well, it tells us where we are and where we need to be.

If you're only at 10 or 20 per cent then we still have a way to go before you are sufficiently convinced by your healthy beliefs to put them into action. If your conviction is at 50 per cent, then you're sort of sitting on the fence, with one leg metaphorically dangling in one garden and one leg in the other, and we have a little bit of work to do before you're ready to plant both feet firmly in your rational garden.

If your conviction is higher, say 60 or 70 per cent, then we are almost there and you are very, nearly, almost ready to confront your disturbance, to handle your activating event in a whole new way. You may have started confronting it already – in which case, well done you.

What this figure represents are the doubts and objections you are still making to your healthy, rational beliefs. So, if your conviction is at 20 per cent, then 80 per cent of you is still saying, 'Yeah but,' and, 'But, what if,' and we need to deal with those objections. If, however, your conviction is at 50 per cent, then only 50 per cent of you is going, 'Yeah, but,' and we still do need to deal with those objections.[1]

However, if your conviction is edging towards the 70 per cent end of the spectrum, then you're very nearly there, and you probably just have one or two doubts left to deal with.

Wherever you sit on that spectrum, we are going to deal with your objections, no matter how many or how few. And we are going to deal with them with what is known as a 'rational-irrational dialogue', or RID for short.

But, before we move on to what this is and what it entails, we need to deal with one very salient point: You cannot get to 100 per cent. And, if you put yourself at 100 per cent, you're kidding yourself. But, why are you doing that? And how?

It's too unrealistic you see. At 100 per cent, you're being utopian, and it won't really allow you to be you. Aim to finish the exercise I'm about to go through with your conviction in your healthy beliefs standing at 75 per cent or higher, but not at 100 per cent. Any lower than 75 per cent, and you still have doubts and objections to tease out and address. But, if you put yourself at 100 per cent it won't allow for any element of doubt. There is no room for the expression of the healthy negative emotion. At 100 per cent, you either don't care anymore or have become devil-may-care and blasé. Neither of these are, therapeutically speaking, are sound places for you to be.

---

[1] For those of you that remember your *Little Britain*, think of Vicky Pollard saying, 'Yeah but, no but, yeah but, no but,' ad infinitum.

Rational-Irrational Dialogue

Do you talk to yourself? Do you hold conversations with your-self, or rehearse arguments or difficult conversations with others before you actually have them, as a sort of 'dry run', just to make sure you've got all your bases covered? Do you discuss the pros and cons of something with yourself, before arriving at a decision, one way or the other? I'm betting that you do.

We all talk to ourselves in one way or another and to some degree or other. It's an innate human ability that we all have, and one that is now going to be used in a specific and targeted way for a definite purpose.

Some of us hold our conversations with ourselves inter-nally, nice and quiet and in our own heads. And, some of us hold these conversations externally, out loud and sometimes, even, quite loudly. I am in the latter camp, unfortunately. I've lost count of the amount of times I've been having a conversa-tion in what I thought was my head, only to notice someone, or several people, staring at me with concern. It's something I've had to make peace with over the years. I'm often to be found out and about, walking the dog usually, muttering to myself, vocally mulling over decisions, life choices, tricky conversa-tions and, at the time of writing, large portions of this book. But, I don't mind the staring, as I have more or less mastered the art of unconditional self-acceptance. Whether I put this as a 'tick' or a 'cross' in the picture of me is neither here nor there.[2]

---

[2] As a most modern plus, many people have alfresco phone con-versations using their headphones, so I just stick mine in, whether I have my phone on me or not; then I blend in with the crowd, and hope people assume I'm talking to someone else.

The point is; we all talk to ourselves. What follows is an exercise where we use that ability to build even more conviction in your healthy beliefs.

Theo, you see, only believed in his healthy beliefs by about 30 per cent at this stage. Which meant that 70 per cent of him remained unconvinced. While he had felt a small emotional shift in the way he felt about being judged by other people, it wasn't enough to help him feel calm enough, or in control enough, or brave enough to do anything about it. If I asked him to go to a party as a homework assignment at this point, he would probably bottle it.

So, firstly, you're going to read through Theo's rational-irrational dialogue, and then, secondly, you're going to attempt one yourself, either in the spare pages of this chapter, or on several pieces of paper, or in an exercise book if you don't want to deface your book (or are a Kindle reader).

Theo's Rational-Irrational Dialogue

Rational

I would prefer not to be judged by other people, but there is no reason why I must not be; it would be bad if I was judged by other people, but it would not be awful. I would find it difficult to deal with if I was judged by other people, but I know I can stand it; I am not a failure, or an idiot, even if other people judge me, I am a worthwhile, fallible human being.

My conviction in this is at 30%

Irrational

Well, that's fine in theory but in reality, it's a completely different thing. On paper it's very reasonable to look at things this way but, when you actually walk into a room, a party, a bar full of people, then it's real, then people mustn't judge you; I must make a good impression, it's really important to.

Rational

Well, that's two demands right there! You're not exactly helping yourself now, are you? There is no law to say people must not judge you and you cannot guarantee you'll make a good impression. At the moment, you don't even turn up, so you're making no impression at all. Yes, it's nice to make a good impression, and it's nice if people do like you. But, those things don't have to happen.

More importantly, if you look at things that way, you'll actually attend the things you're invited to.

Irrational

But, there's a weight of expectation already. If I start socialising, people will already know what I've been like, so it's even more important that I make a good impression, I have to get it right. I can't have people judge me before I've even walked into the room based on what I've been like before. I've ruined things before I've even got there, everyone will look at me.

Rational

Oh no! People will look at you! (Gasp!) You're right, it is important, but it's not the be all and end all. It's simply not true that you have to get this right, you could create a bad impression even if you tried your hardest not to. When you hold a demand like that you are going to put yourself under pressure, and the pressure will show, so you will be less likely to make a good impression. But, when you accept that you don't have to make a good impression even though you want to, you take the pressure off, which allows you to be your natural, authentic self.

Irrational

But, I haven't been my natural, authentic self for years, I'm a loser; I've got nothing to offer.

Rational

You know what? That's bullshit. You are your natural

authentic self when you are on your own and when you are with small groups of friends. They like you, so you can't be a loser. Can I also point out that you're being a bit hypocritical here? You are already judging yourself whilst at the same time demanding that other people do not judge you. You will find it daunting walking into a party or a bar, but not everyone will be out to get you. Some people will like you, some people won't and others may even be indifferent. The important thing here is that you like and accept yourself. When you do that, you are free to focus on the people that do like you.

Irrational

But, it's just like being at school. It's a popularity contest. I failed then and I will fail now. I wasn't popular at school, I was bullied, it was awful then and it will be awful now.

Rational

Look, this isn't school. Mostly it's bars full of people that just want to be happy or it's parties full of people you already know. No one is going to bully you but, even if they do, it's not awful. School wasn't totally bad; you had a lot of good times. You're missing out on a lot by not socialising, which is way more bad than facing off potential judgement or criticism. If you carry on holding your healthy beliefs, what are you going to do? Stay at home for the rest of your life? When you accept that judgement exists, some of it bad, when you accept that not everyone has to like you, and that it's not the end of the world when they don't, you may not feel amazingly confident, but you will feel confident enough to socialise more than you do, and that's the real goal here, isn't it?

Irrational

But, what if other people think I'm a loser because I come across as nervous? If other people think that, then that's what I am.

Rational

Nervous is one thing, anxious is another. It's perfectly fine to be a bit nervous, most people are when they walk into a room, but they quickly relax and so will you. You don't really know what other people think of you. But, you know what? Even if someone does think you're a loser, even if they are actually unkind enough to say it to your face, that judgement won't kill you. You won't like it if they do judge you, you will feel uncomfortable, and who wouldn't? But, you won't keel over and die just because someone thinks you're a loser. You can survive someone's negative appraisal of you. More importantly, you can disagree with them, you can tell them to fuck off, or outright ignore them. Besides, you talk to plenty of people you have a low opinion of and don't mention it. Do you think they'd really care if they found out that you don't really rate them? How is this really going to be any different? Why should you give a hoot if someone you don't really know, doesn't really like you that much?

Irrational

After that, I don't think I've got any more 'yeah, buts' to add. I can't think of any more objections. I could still say 'shouldn't' and 'awful' and so on, but it sounds kind of weak now, I guess.

Rational

Good, so let's revisit your healthy beliefs: 'I hope people don't judge me, but there is no reason why they mustn't; judgement is bad, but it's not awful; I do find judgement difficult to deal with, but I know I can stand it; I am not a loser, or a failure, even if other people judge me, I am a worthwhile, fallible human being.' How much do you believe in all that now?

My conviction in this is at 80%

Points to Ponder

As you've read through the above rational-irrational dialogue, I am hoping that you've noticed a fair few things.

Firstly, the entire conversation is couched in the language of REBT. Behind every irrational objection, there is an unhealthy belief. So, either the objection must not happen, or it is awful, or it is unbearable, or it means that you're a failure in some way. This allows you to espouse the healthy alternative on the rational side of the conversation.

Also, Theo uses the tools of CBT. Disputing is in there, and he's either challenging the validity of the objection and its attendant belief (is it true?) or testing the logic of it (does it make sense?) or pointing out what it does (does it help me?). He also uses persuasion to highlight exactly what the objection and its belief achieve. (He's also used a little bit of swearing to add some force and energy to his counter-arguments – more on that later.)

In essence, whenever you attempt a rational-irrational dialogue you are using everything you have learnt already to effect an increase in your conviction, to increase how much you believe in your healthy beliefs.

In some books, this rational-irrational dialogue is also known as a Zig-Zag Form, as the rational side of the conversation is held on the left hand side of the page, and the irrational side of the conversation is held on the right hand side of the page – with arrows pointing from one side of the conversation to the other, left to right and right to left, zig-zagging down the page until you've run out of conclusions. Like so:

Rational

I'd prefer it if other people didn't get in my way but, there's no reason why they mustn't. It's bad when they get in my way but it isn't awful; I find it difficult to deal with when they get in my way, but I know I can stand it; they're not pillocks, even when they do get in my way, they're worthwhile, fallible human beings.

My conviction: 20%

Irrational

Are you kidding me? I mean, how hard is it to look where you're going? How can you not see that you are about to crash into someone or that you are standing in the doorway of a really busy shop? They are intolerable pillocks, the lot of 'em.

Rational

That's a bit harsh isn't it? No wonder you explode. It's not intolerable. You're not going to die or explode just because someone bumps into you; you will survive the occasion. And, they're not pillocks they're worthwhile, fallible human beings, doing their best to deal with a crowded situation, just like you are.

If you read other books on REBT, as well as a Zig-Zag Form, the dialogue is also sometimes called an 'attack-defence exercise' as, instead of the term 'rational' for the rational side of the conversation, you use the word 'defence', and instead of the word 'irrational' for the unhelpful side of the conversation, you use the term 'attack'.[3]

Whatever you want to call it, as you go through the exercise yourself, don't assume that just because you have addressed an objection, the objection has been dealt with, as objections don't tend to go away without a fair bit of sulking and skulking around first.

---

[3] And far too many people over the years have called it the 'yeah but no but' exercise, with 'yeah but' standing for the rational and 'no but' standing for the irrational.

I'm sure you've all had one of those conversations with a child. The one where they ask you something, or object to something, and you give them a very well-rounded and well-reasoned response. They pause for a moment, digesting what you have just said, and then reply with, 'But why?'

So, you sigh, and give them another well-reasoned response. And, again, they ask, 'But why?' And again, and again, and again until you give up and shout back, 'Because, I bloody well said so, that's why!'

Your objections will be a lot like those little children. You'll formulate a well-rounded and well-reasoned rational response, but your objection will remain the same, or be nearly the same, or will say the same thing in a slightly different way. It will still be asking, 'But why?' And you will have to reason with it again, and again until it is either dealt with, or until you shout out, 'Because I bloody well said so, that's why!'

How to Construct a Rational-Irrational Dialogue

1. Write the word 'rational' and then, underneath that, write down your healthy belief in full.
2. Underneath your healthy belief, rate, as a percentage, how much you believe in your healthy belief and then draw a tiny little arrow going down.
3. Next, write down the word 'irrational' and then write down your first objection to your healthy belief – your first doubt, your first 'yeah but'. And, then write down whatever belief you think lies behind your doubt. Then draw another little arrow going down.

4. Again, write the word 'rational,' indicating that you're back to the rational side of the conversation and, using the language of CBT, your healthy beliefs, the tools of disputing and persuasion, rationalise your objection. Then draw a little arrow going down . . .

5. Now, write the word 'irrational' and write down another objection, again noting down which of the four unhealthy beliefs you think lie behind that objection. Then draw a little arrow going down.

6. Keeping going, from the rational to the irrational, from a doubt and an objection to a rational and emotive response to that doubt or objection.

7. Keep going. Keep responding in kind. Put down all your doubts and objections and keep rationalising them out using what you have learnt from REBT so far, and how you think, feel and act when you are endorsing the unhealthy points and how you think, feel and act when you are endorsing the healthy points. Keep going until you have run out of doubts and objections.

8. Don't just complete one side of A4 paper or one page of this book. This may take one, two, three or more sheets of paper. Try and increase your arguments and dialogues in complexity as you go along.[4]

---

[4] The biggest dialogue I ever received as a piece of homework from a client was a real doozy: 48 pages long and full of well-reasoned responses, opinions from family and friends, quick quips and comebacks, words of wisdom, poems, song lyrics, quotes and pictures. But, don't be afraid, as yours does not have to be this involved.

9. When you finish, bring your dialogue back round to your healthy beliefs and, finally, rate your conviction as a percentage in your healthy beliefs again. The idea being that, as you go along, you are endorsing the healthy point of view, arguing consistently, rationally and persuasively in favour of your healthy beliefs, and increasing your conviction from beginning to end.

10. Run through this exercise over and again, in your head and out loud, using some of the fundamental arguments you have used, to take control of your thoughts, feelings and behaviours in the appropriate situations.

11. I hope this all made sense, so it's time to grab paper and pen.

'But,' I hear you cry, 'that's a lot of writing things down and I feel I've written enough things down already. I need a bit of a writing break.'

To which I say, 'Teddy bears'.

Talking to Stuffed Toys

Every course I've even been on has required that I practice, practice, practice – just like you are being asked to do in this chapter – to not only get used to the tools of REBT, but to effect that shift from one way of thinking to the other.

As a student, I've not always had a person to practice on. I've lost count of how many times over the years, as I studied and practised, that I've put a teddy bear in a chair and either hypnotised it (practising not only how to hypnotise someone in a variety of ways, with different techniques, but also how to treat certain conditions and emotional problems), or practised disputing, or rehearsed persuasive arguments, or engaged in a rational-irrational dialogue.[5]

So, if you've got a teddy bear yourself, or some other stuffed animal for that matter, or a doll or an anything, put it in a chair and talk to it. Obviously, you're engaging in both sides of the conversation and you may want to adopt a slightly different tone, or even a silly voice for the irrational side of the conversation. Plenty of people have tried it this way over the years, and to good effect. It's not as silly as it sounds and can be quite cathartic.

But, if you don't like the idea of talking to your teddy bear, or you're worried that someone might come in and catch you, there's always the voice memo function on your smartphone, which you may have already used for the disputing exercise or persuasive arguments.

The handy thing here is that, once you've gone through your rational-irrational dialogue, you can then play it back as many times as you like to really entrench both the conversation and your conviction in your healthy beliefs. Again, you may want to alter your voice slightly for the irrational side of the conversation and, for added effect, you might also want to pivot slightly from foot to foot as you do so, with the left foot indicating the rational side of the conversation and the right foot indicating the irrational side of the conversation.

Remember your percentages. If, by the time you have finished, your conviction is only at, say, 65 per cent, you still have

---

[5] Oh, the things that bear could tell you. Poor Teddy.

objections to tease out. But, if you are in the high seventies or low eighties, you have done a really good job.

You can't get to 100 per cent as that is both unrealistic and utopian. Anything under that but over 70 means you are ready to put your money where your mouth is. It's time to put what you've written and/or spoken about into practice.

The 'B' in REBT Stands for Behaviour

When your conviction in your healthy beliefs is high enough, you now need to start acting in accordance with those beliefs. You need to start putting things into practice. If you don't, everything you've written thus far is, and will remain, theoretical. Now, your homework assignments become behavioural.

For instance, armed with my healthy beliefs of 'I prefer it when other people don't get in my way, but there is no reason why they mustn't; it's bad when other people get in my way, but it is not awful; I find it difficult to deal with when other people get in my way, but I know I can stand it; and the people who get in my way are not complete idiots, they are worthwhile fallible human beings' and a conviction rate of 85 per cent, I was ready to go back into crowded spaces. Not just occasionally, but repeatedly: again and again, until I felt a shift in my emotions, until I felt in control of the situation and myself.

So, I took myself off to places where lots of people congregated and I did so as often as possible: public transport at rush hour, train platforms at the same time, shopping centres at the weekend, popular bars and clubs, you name it; anywhere and everywhere that would test me until I could safely say that, to all intents and purposes, I was merely frustrated in crowded places, rather than angry.

Theo meanwhile, armed with an 80 per cent conviction rate in the healthy beliefs he knew would help him achieve his goals, had to socialise as much as possible, as often as possible. He recited his healthy beliefs and referred to the homework if needed until, like me, to all intents and purposes, he could safely say that he was nervous when socialising, but no longer anxious. And, I say referring to the homework if needed, because sometimes that's what you need to do; that's what it's there for.

Over the years, I've had many people put their homework on their smartphones and tablets, to keep them to hand. If you feel you need a little refresher in the moment, if you feel like your disturbance is trying to wrestle back control, it's very easy to nip to the loo and use your exercises to get yourself back under control (and plenty of people have, and continue to do so).

So, what have you been working on as you've gone through this book and how will you test how well you've been doing?

For instance, if it's a dog phobia you're working on, you will need to expose yourself to as many dogs as you can. If you're depressed at the direction your life has taken and have disengaged with life, now is the time to reengage with it as much as you can. If, like I had, you have an anger-management issue, you need to expose yourself to the anger-provoking situation, or person, repeatedly; and if, like Theo, yours is a social anxiety problem, then you will need to make yourself quite the social butterfly over the next few weeks and months. You can even have a few dry runs first using just your imagination.

In REBT, and other cognitive behavioural therapies, any behavioural assignments you are set, or that you set yourself can be conducted either *in vivo* or *in vitro*.

Putting yourself into a situation *in vivo* means doing it for real, as it means 'real life'. So, that would involve me actively going to a crowded shopping mall and it would involve Theo actively going to a party. But, *in vitro* means doing the same thing, only with your imagination. This would involve me sitting in a chair, eyes closed, imagining myself in crowded places, imagining people bumping into me and tripping over me, while reciting my healthy beliefs and thinking and feeling and acting according to those beliefs. And it would be the same for Theo, sitting in a chair, eyes closed only imagining himself at the party, reciting his healthy beliefs while imagining some negative judgement, and acting in accordance with his healthy beliefs. This is a surprisingly effective technique.

Some people prefer to jump straight into doing it for real, while some prefer a few dry runs in their imagination first.

If you start off *in vitro*, you will have to move it up to *in vivo* at some point though and, with both techniques, repetition is key. And don't worry if all doesn't go according to plan immediately, that's what all the previous homework is for. Use the homework, read through it wherever you are and whenever you need it. Use it to take control of your emotions and behaviours.

If you did well in your behavioural assignment, make a note of it. If you did good; but not as well as you would like to, make a note of it. More importantly, if you returned to form; if you got anxious, or depressed, or angry, make a note of what you said that had you feeling like that and add it to the rational-irrational dialogue. Work on it and rationalise it out and then test yourself again.

The idea here is to keep going. The more you repeat your healthy beliefs and the more you act in accordance with your healthy beliefs, the more you are fixing the habit of thinking and feeling and acting like a whole new you, a healthy and rational you. Hence the title of this chapter, 'repeat, repeat, repeat'. (If any Doctor Who fans are reading this book, please feel free to say it like a Dalek if you want to. Believe me when I say, many people have.)

Stuff to Do for Week Five

- Construct your rational-irrational dialogue and build up your conviction in your healthy beliefs as high as possible (there is space on the next page). Read through it and rehearse it a fair few times.
- When you feel you are ready, initiate as many behavioural assignments as you can, either in your imagination, or for real, or both.
- Note down your successes, your near misses and the times it went wrong (if indeed it did at all). If it did go wrong, note down what you said that had you returning to previous behaviours and add it to your rational-irrational dialogue.
- Keep practising.

Before you start the chapter on Week Six, answer the following reflective questions:

257

Reflective Questions

- What is this chapter about and how have you applied that knowledge?
- What behavioural assignments have you tried? How pleased are you with your progress? If you're not as pleased as you would like to be, what do you think is hampering your progress?
- Have you had any insights or 'light bulb' moments as a result of reading through this chapter, in challenging your beliefs this way, in putting it into practice and in reflecting on what other areas they may relate to over the past week?

Your Rational-Irrational Dialogue:

Your behavioural assignments are . . .

. . . In vivo	. . . In vitro

Week Six

Putting the 'Fun' into 'Dysfunctional'

My mission in life is not merely to survive, but to thrive; and to do so with some passion, some compassion, some humour and some style.

Maya Angelou

How do you feel as a result of all the work you have undertaken so far? How close do you feel to the full achievement of your goal? I'm hoping you feel nearly there or, better still, very nearly there.

Do you want something to get you right there? You do? Well, that's good then. Here goes.

Earlier in this book I mentioned that, in a 1982 professional survey of US and Canadian psychologists, Albert Ellis was widely considered to be the second most influential psychotherapist in history, with Freud coming in at number three.

The person that took the number one position was American psychologist Carl Rogers. A founding father of the humanistic (or client-centred) approach to therapy, among his many accolades, achievements and works were the development of what are now called the 'core conditions'. These are attributes that a counsellor or therapist had to possess, or needed to display, in order to help the person in his, hers or their therapy room.

These core conditions have been widely accepted, not just by humanistic therapists, but also by pretty much all therapists, no matter their discipline or background. There are three core conditions: empathy, congruence and unconditional positive regard.

Empathy means being able to understand things from the client's perspective, (walking in their shoes, so to speak). Congruence means being genuine and real, (which helps build trust and rapport). Finally, we have unconditional positive regard, which is the ability to allow the client to speak about anything they feel they need to without fear of being judged or criticised (very important if they are going to trust you with their deepest, darkest secrets).

Rogers considered these core conditions both 'necessary and sufficient'. By that, he meant that they needed to be in place for therapeutic change to occur (necessary) and that, if they were in place, therapeutic change would occur (sufficient).

However, Albert Ellis disagreed. He considered these conditions neither necessary nor sufficient. While he believed that change would be more likely to take place if they were in place, he also believed that change could occur even if they were not. And, as if to prove a point, Albert Ellis himself could be a fairly prickly individual who did not score very highly on ratings of warmth or empathy, and yet he was a highly successful therapist.

He also added a fourth core condition, namely humour.

Part of the problem, said Ellis, was not that clients were taking themselves, or others, or world conditions seriously, but that they were taking them far too seriously indeed. He believed that if you could help them lighten up, or even laugh at their beliefs and the disturbances they caused, then you would have helped them greatly in the process of change.

'Why not poke the blokes with jolly jokes,' he said. 'Or split their shit with wit.'[1]

To that end he would introduce jokes, puns, witticisms, slang, absurdity, obscene language and more into the therapy room. Not to attack the client directly, not to criticise them in any way, but to ridicule, demean and laugh at their unhealthy beliefs and the crazy ideas they produced.

I wrote my MSc dissertation on the use of humour in psychotherapy, so I'm a big fan of getting people to laugh at some of the thoughts they have in their heads. Someone must have found my thesis funny, because it got published in a journal.

It's not for nothing that laughter is called the best medicine, and the benefits of it are numerous and well documented. Laughter triggers healthy physical changes in the body. Humour and laughter strengthen your immune system, boost your energy, diminish pain and protect you from the damaging effects of stress. They protect the heart and trigger the release of endorphins (the body's natural feel-good chemicals). Mentally they increase wellbeing, reduce stress, improve mood, enhance resilience and improve relationships. They literally help you stay emotionally healthy.

Studies have shown that laughter can dissolve distressing emotions (it's hard to feel anxious or depressed when you're laughing); that it helps you relax and recharge and helps you shift perspective, so you literally see situations and problems in a more realistic and less threatening light. It can also create psychological distance, helping you to avoid feeling overwhelmed. Humour and playful communication can strengthen our relationships by triggering positive feelings and fostering an emotional connection too.

With all that in mind, who wouldn't want to bring some more funny stuff into their lives? To that end, this is the chapter where you will swear, sing songs and shout out your favourite movie quotes; not for the sheer hell of it (although that is fun), but to effect a change in the way you think, feel and act.

A very good way of making a shift from one way of thinking to another is to not just dispute your beliefs, but to dispute them vigorously and repeatedly. It also helps to shout or yell your beliefs (out loud or in your head) with force and energy.

And a really, really good way of adding force and energy to your arguments is by swearing.

Seriously, tell your unhealthy beliefs to just fuck off. It's not for nothing that the F-bomb is built into the very title of this book.

Many studies have backed up the usefulness of swearing in a variety of settings. Swearing can help you cope with adversity, get on with people more quickly, cope with difficult and demanding situations and, here's the important bit, bolster the persuasiveness of your arguments.

---

[1] Perhaps indicating that Albert wasn't quite as funny as he liked to think he was.

One such experiment, from researchers at Northern Illinois University, examined the effects of swearing on the persuasiveness of a speech. Participants were invited to listen to three versions of a speech. One where the word 'damn' appeared at the beginning, one where it appeared at the end and one where it didn't appear at all. The results showed that swearing at the beginning or the end of the speech significantly increased not only the persuasiveness of the speech but also the perceived intensity of the speaker.[2]

Meanwhile, Professor Richard Stephens over at Keele University has tested swearing in a wide variety of ways over the years. He and his team discovered that people who swear can hold their hands in freezing cold water for longer than those who don't swear and that, in a test of anaerobic strength, people who swore produced more power wattage and a stronger handgrip on a stationary exercise bike than those who did not. He and his team even discovered that men who exhibited the tendency to catastrophise (i.e. do a drama) had less tolerance to pain, even when they swore.

Swearing is a great way to gain control, not only over your pain and stress, but also of your emotions. So, in short, if you want to improve the power of your persuasive arguments or, if you want to give your healthy beliefs more of a kick in crunchtime moments, don't be afraid to drop the F-bomb.

---

[2] In what is possibly the only academic reference in this book: Cory R. Scherer and Brad J. Sagarin (2006) 'Indecent influence: The positive effects of obscenity on persuasion', *Social Influence*, 1:2, 138–146

In fact, if you do swear, it's going to become part of your homework for this week.

Elsewhere, studies have shown that people who swear (as long as swearing is part of their overall extensive vocabulary) tend to be healthier, happier and a whole lot more honest too.

But, what about its effects with Rational Emotive Behaviour Therapy?

Let's say you have a drug addiction. In terms of unhealthy beliefs, the addiction is easy to understand (not the reasons for doing your thing and becoming addicted in the first place, which can be many and varied), but the language of your brain expecting and, indeed, anticipating the next hit of the happy-happy stuff. It's your brain going, 'I must have my thing, gimme, gimme, gimme! I can't cope another minute without my hit.' And it's going to be saying it very loudly and very strongly, while giving you massive urges to do your drug of choice.

The healthy, rational and helpful alternative to that is this, 'I would like to have my thing, but I don't have to have it; saying no to my thing will be difficult, but I know I can stand it'.

Do you think that will be enough to stave off the urge to use whatever it is that you've become addicted to? It might, if you have disputed your beliefs vigorously and repeatedly enough, but how about this for a belief:

'SURE, I'D LIKE TO HAVE MY THING, BUT I DON'T FUCKING HAVE TO HAVE IT; SAYING NO WILL BE HARD BUT IT WON'T FUCKING KILL ME!'

It has more 'oomph', don't you think? Now say it louder. Now shout it out as loud as you can. How do you feel? Do you feel all, 'Hell yeah!'

Now we're talking.

For instance, Theo liked swearing. Hopefully, you're very familiar with his healthy beliefs by now. When he added force and energy (i.e. swearing) to them, they looked like this:

'I hope people don't judge me, but they can do what the fuck they like; judgement is bad, but it's not the worst fucking thing to happen; I don't like it and I don't fucking have to but it won't fucking kill me; there is nothing fucking wrong with me, I am fucking fine'.

There are other colourful ways to add force and energy to your beliefs: song lyrics, movie quotes, your favourite movie scene or passage from a book. And, you can even add swearing to them for extra effect.

One client of mine was addicted to crystal meth. It's a drug that can exert quite the strong grip if you're not careful. His healthy non-drug taking belief was very similar to the above, plus he was also self-damning (I am weak because I want to use it) and we were working on his self-acceptance (I'm not weak, even though I want my thing; I am a worthwhile fallible human being). It was helping, but it wasn't quite enough to pass muster or curb his usage.

My client was a 'Ringer' (a fan of the works of J. R. R Tolkien in general and a fan of *The Lord of the Rings* trilogy specifically). To cut a very long and awesome story short for people who have no idea what *The Lord of the Rings* is about: there is a very bad sorcerer called Sauron and he forged one very powerful ring for himself, a ring that enhanced all his evil powers. But, and here's the really naughty bit, he also created several rings for the elves, the dwarves and the kings of men, as gifts and under the pretext of friendship. What he didn't tell them was that the rings were secretly in thrall to and controlled by his one ring. The elves and the dwarves, more or less, looked at the rings and went, 'Pfft.' However, the nine kings of men said, 'Ooh, shiny, thank you,' and put on the rings. They very quickly fell from grace and became 'Ringwraiths'. They were ghosts, shadows of their former selves and slaves to the one ring and its master.

And this is how my client described himself on the very first session, a Ringwraith, a ghost, a shadow, and a slave to his drug. He'd be in a bar, or at a party, and all the people around him were alive and vibrant, while he felt like an apparition.

There is also a good and powerful wizard in *The Lord of the Rings* by the name of Gandalf. You can tell he is a wizard, because he has a wizard's staff. There is a particularly powerful scene in the book where Gandalf is on a bridge over a great chasm, trying to protect his friends from an approaching giant fire demon called a Balrog. As the Balrog tries to cross the bridge, Gandalf bellows, 'You cannot pass!' He then smashes his staff down on the bridge, breaking the bridge to pieces, and pummels the demon with magical energy, casting it into the abyss.[3]

It's such a popular and stirring passage from the book that not only did it appear at the end of the first in the trilogy of movies, but director Peter Jackson saw fit to repeat it to kick off the second movie in the trilogy. Although, in the movie, Gandalf yells, 'You shall not pass,' instead of, 'You cannot pass.'

I discussed adding force and energy and swearing with my client and suggested he added these to his beliefs and monitor the results. We also discussed movies and books and songs.

---

[3] From whence it came. Everyone in a Tolkien novel has to say 'From whence it came' at least once.

When he returned the next week, he nervously handed me a piece of paper. On it he had written, 'I am not a fucking Ringwraith, I am fucking Gandalf!'

Over the course of the previous week, every time he experienced the urge to use his drug he shouted this phrase either in his head or out loud. He also imagined himself as Gandalf, on that bridge and screaming out, 'You shall not pass!' Then bashing his metaphorical staff on his meta-phorical bridge and blasting his actual urge to use with metaphorical magical energy, thereby casting his particular demon into the abyss.[4]

He then asked me if he'd done the homework correctly, which he had, because he reported the best week he'd had so far and went on to successfully remain clean from the last session to this.

So, if you want to swear your fucking beliefs going for-wards, I will support the shit out of your fucking decision.

But, what do you do if you don't like swearing? Well, you don't have to swear if you don't want to, as there's more than one way to be emotive. If you don't swear, but you do use words such as 'fudge' and 'fiddlesticks' in their place then, by all means, use them.[5]

'I would like to be on time for everything,' you could say, 'But, I don't fudging have to.' Or whatever, your particular beliefs are. Now say them louder. And again. Now shout them out really loud. Louder still. How do you feel?

---

[4] From whence it came, obviously.

[5] I have a friend and had clients who do indeed use these as swear-words.

I'm hoping you feel good, I'm hoping you feel empowered.

More than a few clients over the years have turned their beliefs into something like this: 'Oh for crying out loud Sarah, other people do not have to do what you want even though you want them to. You don't like it and you don't have to like it but, for the love of all that is holy, you've got this. You can deal with it.' Statements such as these are true to the spirit of REBT, are passionate and empowering and yet do not contain any swearwords at all.

But, back to *The Lord of the Rings*, and to books in general.

Movies and literature are a great source of inspiration. We all have favourite scenes, favourite moments, favourite quotes. If you do, use them. Over the years many Harry Potter fans have turned their beliefs into spells and charms that mirror their favourite parts of either the books or the movies. More than a fair few clients have just effectively poured everything they've learnt into an 'expelliarmus' or a 'riddikulus' and, even, an 'expecto patronum'. The latter incantation complete with attendant image of a full-blown 'patronus' of their choice.

Plus, I have it on good authority that 'expecto fucking patronum' really does work like a charm on dispelling not only unhealthy beliefs, but, also, the disturbing emotions and behaviours they produce.

Songs work too. Often our favourite song lyrics can become quite symbolic of the REBT process, the very words become synonymous with the healthy beliefs you are working on.

Another one of my clients presented with an anger-management issue. Especially when things weren't going his way, or when he felt stupid, belittled or demeaned in any way. He was a big, burly chap. When it came round to discussing adding force and energy to, not only his beliefs, but to his persuasive arguments, I discussed swearing, but he shook his head vigorously.

'Please don't make me swear,' he said. 'I've got two young daughters. I've had to work really hard at not swearing and I don't want to start again.'

'That's okay,' I said. 'No swearing then.' And I discussed movies, books and songs. His homework was to come up with something that he found empowering that gave his beliefs a little bit of kick.

He came back a week later and, when I asked if had come up with something, he looked a little sheepish.

'Well, I did do it,' he said.

'Good,' I said. 'What did you develop?'

'Well, I've got two young girls, haven't I?'

I nodded, 'Go on,' I said.

'They love that movie. *Frozen*. Do you know it?'

I did know it. And I knew where this was going.

'They play it over and over again. They make me sing along with them sometimes. There's this one song–'

You know the one. I know the one. He didn't need to say any more. Every time he started to feel angry, he sang 'Let it Go'.

Courtesy of his daughters and their love of *Frozen*, every single word of that main song, the big number, had become indelibly etched upon his mind and had, oddly, become quite synonymous with the healthy beliefs we had been working on. And he was indeed singing the song every time he started to lose his temper. In his head, obviously, not out loud.

'Did it work?' I asked

'Oh yes,' he said. 'It's been great.'

Over the years, as I've shared this therapeutic anecdote, many people have returned to my clinic saying, 'Actually, 'Let it Go' works for me too. I've not been able to get that song out of my head. And it's really helped.' I have no idea how many people are now out there singing this song from *Frozen* as a way of encapsulating their beliefs.[6]

It may sound strange but songs really do help. They empower, they enable and they allow you to cope with adversity.

Who here hasn't staggered around their bedroom or living room, clutching a half-drunk bottle of wine, while belting out a break-up ballad to power their way through the emotions of a recently failed relationship?[7]

So you can swear your beliefs, you can shout your beliefs, you can attach book and movie moments and quotes to your beliefs, and you can sing songs about your beliefs. Be careful with the songs though, as most songs are bonkers (and, by bonkers, I mean they are replete with irrational language). Allow me to elaborate.

Irrational Language in Songs

Sadly irrational language surrounds us. We hear other people speak it, we speak it; we think it and feel it. It's on our

---

[6] 'Let It Go' comes courtesy of husband-and-wife songwriting team Kristen Anderson-Lopez and Robert Lopez and was sung by actress and singer Idina Menzel. If only they knew what wonders their song had wrought in therapy. Someone tell them, please.

[7] 'Weak', by Skunk Anansie, if you're asking.

televisions and it's in our books and, if you listen to music, it is most definitely in our songs, especially in our love songs and our torch songs.

When it comes to love and relationships, most lyrics are very irrational indeed. We all know how love songs tend to go. Whether they are in a pop, dance, rock or blues vein, and whether it's some delicate strings or a thumping base that accompanies them, they tend to go a lot like this . . .

> *I have to have you*
> *You have to love me*
> *There's you and only you*
> *Woah, woah, woah*
> *Love, love, love*
> *I can't stand life without you*
> *Life's not worth living without you*
> *I'll never find love again*
> *Woah, woah, woah*
> *Love, love, love*

Well, when spun through the REBT machine, lyrics such as those above tend to look a lot like this . . .

> *I would like to have you, but I don't have to have you*
> *And I would like you to love me, but you don't have to*
>   *love me*
> *There's someone else out there who will reciprocate my*
>   *feelings*
> *Woah, woah, woah*
> *Love, love, love*

272

> *I might find it difficult to deal with if I don't have you, but I*
> *   can cope with that*
> *I will find other things in life enjoyable in the meantime*
> *And, eventually, fall in love with someone else*
> *Woah, woah, woah*
> *Love, love, love*

Okay, so lyrics like that will not a hit record make, but they are going to introduce some sanity into the proceedings. Which is needed because, let's face it, love is not the most rational of emotions. Take 'All You Need is Love' by The Beatles, for instance. Do you? Is love all that you need? Do you even need it at all?

In 1943, psychologist Abraham Maslow outlined a human hierarchy of needs in his paper 'A Theory of Human Motivation'. Essentially, this hierarchy is a pyramid comprised of five layers of need: physiological, safety, belonging/love, esteem and self-actualisation. Of the five, only the bottom layer, made up of food, water, warmth and rest were 'must haves', in that, without them, you would die (either quickly or slowly, depending on the need). All other needs in Maslow's pyramid are preferential. While you might not like life without them, you will live. So, with Maslow in mind, All You Need is Love (a tier-three need) becomes:

> *Love is nice to have, but you don't have to have it (repeat,*
> *   repeat)*
> *Love, love, love*
> *Love is preferable*

While rational, it's now rendered rubbish as a love song, but, it was definitely the sort of thing Albert Ellis would sing either to or with his clients.

So, let's see if you can spot the original love songs from the rational lyrics below. Answers at the end of the chapter if you can't but, first up, there's this:

> *I will find it difficult to deal with, but I know I can live*
> *If living is without you*
> *I may not feel like giving again initially, but I will heal, recover, move on*
> *And give again, but to someone else*

Secondly, how about this one?

> *Tell me, tell me baby*
> *Why can't you leave me?*
> *'Cause even though I wish I didn't want it, I do*
> *I would like to have it, but I don't have to have it*
> *I would like to have you, you, you, but I don't have to have you, you, you*

The final one, however, might be a bit of a giveaway . . .

> *Girl's name, girl's name, girl's name, girl's name*
> *I'm politely asking you not to take my man*
> *Girl's name, girl's name, girl's name, girl's name*
> *I would prefer it if you didn't even though there's no law to say you mustn't*

Most love songs contain more than their fair share of 'should nots' and 'got tos', as well as 'awfuls' and 'unbearables'. Which ain't good. Sadly, while rational language is great for keeping you calm and sane, even when going through a painful break-up, or dealing with a cheating lover, it does make for some really rubbish lyrics that no decent songster or songstress is ever going to want to belt out anthem-style.

Part of your homework will be to seek out an irrational love song, and rewrite the lyrics, so that they become much more in keeping with the teachings of REBT.

Rational Language in Songs

As an added bonus, you can even go looking for a rational love song, if you want. Because, they do exist: they are just few and far between. Even 'Let it Go' from *Frozen* has its fair share of irrationality, but you can't go wrong rationally with 'Que Sera, Sera' by Doris Day or 'You Can't Always Get What You Want' by The Rolling Stones.

Believe me, I've set homework assignments such as these with plenty of people I see for therapy and we've had lots of fun doing so. One guy even translated a period German aria into English and then turned it into a rational song.

Moving away from the world of music, however, and back to normal, everyday, irrational language. When people hold unhealthy beliefs, they think, feel and act irrationally. They speak irrationally and their language affects how they think, feel and act. Take the following passage, from a lady who had a work-related stress problem:

'The problem is my boss. I can't stand her. She's a total fucking nightmare. She makes my life hell. She makes all our lives hell. She's all right outside of work, but at work she's a cow, a complete fucking cow. One minute she's all sweetness and light, the next minute she talks to your like you're filth. Some of her emails are reasonable and some of them are crazy. And there's no rhyme or reason to it. You never know how she is going to behave, or what she's going to do next. She is literally Jekyll and Hyde. It makes work-life unbearable. Everyone's on tenterhooks. It drives me fucking crazy. She shouldn't be like that. She should have more respect for her staff. It fucks me off. It's terrible the way she treats us. She makes me anxious and angry. I bottle it up. I come home most days feeling like a right failure, worrying about how I will cope with what the next day brings. I'm cracking up I am.'

Now, having read the above:

- How do you think this person feels?
- How do you think they act at work?
- What do they likely do when they get home from work?
- How do they deal with their boss?

Rational Language

I would like you to rewrite the above passage, using everything you have learnt so far, by using the principles of REBT and the role of healthy beliefs in psychological wellbeing. If you struggle, I've written a more rational version of the above conversation on the next page. But, have a go first. Don't peek.

You peeked, didn't you?

A More Rational Version

'I'm having a problem with my boss. She can be a bit difficult to deal with sometimes. At times she can be a bit nasty. She can be a real challenge sometimes, not just for me, but for everybody. She's all right outside of work, but at work she's not always very pleasant. One minute she's all sweetness and light, the next minute she talks down to you. Some of her emails are reasonable and some of them aren't very reasonable at all. And there's no rhyme or reason to it. You never know how she is going to behave, or what she's going to do next. You know that book, *Dr Jekyll and Mr Hyde*? She reminds of that. I know I can deal with her, even though she is challenging and rude at times, I'm just not sure I want to. Everyone's on tenterhooks. It's not the most enjoyable environment to be in. I don't know why she is like it, I wish she wasn't, but sadly she is. I mean, I'm no angel myself sometimes but, it would be nice if she treated her staff with more respect. I know she doesn't have to; it's not awful or anything like that, but it is very unpleasant. Dealing with her can be frustrating, and wondering how she will be brings an added pressure. I don't bottle it up or anything, but I do come home more tired and stressed than I would like to be. It's a shame, because I love the actual job and I'm very good at it. Staying means dealing with her on a daily basis, but going means losing a job I enjoy. I guess I'd like to give less of a fuck about her and her attitude. Yes, that would be nice. Then I could decide what I want to do.'

Having written your own version or read the above . . .

- How does this person feel?
- How do they act at work?
- What do they do when away from work?
- How do they deal with their boss?

But, what does this mean for the problem you have been working on and the beliefs behind them?

Well, for the following week and onwards, I want you to swear your beliefs, or sing songs or recall movie quotes and passages of book, and even all of the above, as you go through the situations you have been putting yourself in.

That's the important bit: Keep doing those behavioural assignments. Keep putting yourself in those situations that you found problematic. Or dealing with the people that you found difficult. And do so while reciting your healthy beliefs (with added force and energy) and monitoring your results.

For instance, Theo found that if he felt a little anxiety rising at a party or social gathering (he went to the pub twice and to a small house party) then swearing his healthy beliefs brought an immediate sense of relief and, more importantly, an immediate sense of control. This, coupled with the progress he'd experienced in the previous week's homework, meant that he felt that his goal had been achieved and that he was happy for this to be his last session with me. He felt confident, he felt like that he had 'got this'.

You've Got This Too

And there you have it: six weeks and six steps through the REBT process, following the ABCDE model of psychological health while working on one particular problem. You have learnt how to hang a problem off that model and, in doing so, have discovered how to pick a problem, identify the unhealthy emotion attached to that problem and then worked out the aspect of the problem that disturbs you the most.

From there, you have correctly identified your unhealthy beliefs and then formulated the healthy equivalents to those beliefs. After that, you disputed your beliefs, developed persuasive arguments that looked at what your unhealthy beliefs were getting you and what your healthy beliefs could get you. Then, having built a measure of conviction in your healthy beliefs, you strengthened that conviction by dealing with any and all doubts and objections using a rational-irrational dialogue.

Finally, you have added force and energy to both your beliefs by adding swearing and songs and movie snippets. All to effect a shift in the way you think, feel and act in the face of the problem you picked to work on.

I hope you are happy with the results.

This places you at 'E' in the ABCDE model. It means that, if everything has gone according to plan, you now have an effective rational outlook on that original activating event. But, what happens now? What comes next and how do you maintain your gains in the weeks, months and years to come?

All that is covered in the next chapter but, before that, there is the small matter of some homework to attend to.

Stuff to Do for Week Six

- If you swear, add swearwords to your beliefs and/or your rational-irrational dialogue and your persuasive arguments. If you don't swear, turn your beliefs into songs. Or do both. Both is good.
- Carry on with your behavioural assignments, in your imagination or for real, or both, using force and energy to add extra conviction in times of need.
- Note down your successes, your near-misses and the times it went wrong (if indeed it did at all).
- Keep practising.
- Find an irrational song and rewrite it, using everything that you have learnt, so that it is now a rational song.

Before you read the next chapter, answer the following reflective questions.

Reflective Questions

- What is this chapter about and how have you applied that knowledge?
- What behavioural assignments have you tried? How pleased are you with your progress? What has adding force and energy to your beliefs and arguments brought you in terms of improvement?
- What irrational song did you find? What do you think of the rational version? Do any songs remind

you of the work you have been doing on your healthy beliefs. If so, which ones and why?

- Have you had any insights or 'light bulb' moments as a result of reading through this chapter, in challenging your beliefs this way, in putting it into practice and in reflecting on what other areas they may relate to over the past week?

Guess the Song Lyrics

How did you do? Do you think you worked out the original irrational versions of the rational love songs? First up, we had 'Without You', originally performed by Welsh rock band Badfinger in 1970 (written by Pete Ham and Tom Evans), but also made famous by Air Supply and Mariah Carey. This was followed by 'Problem', which was a 2014 hit from Ariana Grande featuring Iggy Azalea (written by Ariana Grande, Iggy Azalea, Ilya, Max Martin and Sava Kotecha). Finally, we had Dolly Parton and her 1973 classic, 'Jolene'.

What Now?

The only real problem in life is what to do next.

Arthur C Clarke

If you have worked through your problem, we are now firmly at the 'E' in the ABCDE model of psychological health. E stands for an Effective rational outlook on that original activating event. It can also mean the end of work on that problem. Sort of.

I say sort of because change is a life-long process. And so is any form of therapy, including REBT, but don't worry, that's really not as scary as it sounds.

If you were seeing me for therapy, not only could E mean an effective rational outlook to the problem you were working on, but it could also mean the end of work on that problem and the beginning of work on the next. You could do that too; if you have found this book helpful on working on one par-ticular emotional problem, there's no reason why you can't go through the same process again on another one.

E can also mean The End of therapy, but that ending is never as final as it seems. Some people like a short and sharp end; problem solved, goal achieved, bye-bye and out the door – an 'I don't need to see you unless I need to see you' sort of thing. For others, it's a more gradual, tapered-off kind of ending, spreading sessions out over a few weeks or a few months, monitoring their progress, not only in maintaining their gains on the problem or problems that we worked on, but also on how effective it has been on other areas of their life in general.

And that's where we are; that's what comes next. Whether you're reading this book and applying that knowledge for yourself and to yourself, or whether you've finished with any kind of therapist from any kind of discipline. It's all about maintaining your gains.

Many people read self-help books, enjoy them, find meaning in them, then put them back on the shelf and forget all about them. Then they pick up another self-help book and repeat the process. And, you know what happens to those sorts of people, don't you?

But, if a book, or a therapy or a therapist has touched you, moved you, changed you and helped you for the better, then don't you owe it to yourself and to your psychological wellbe-ing to keep that process alive?

Doing that involves a variety of factors that we will go through here.

First of all, if you could sum up what you have learnt from this book in one sentence or as one insight, what would that sentence or insight be?

Everyone is different, for some it's to give up their demands, for others it's to never awfulise or dramatise again; for others still it's the belief that they can cope with anything that life throws at them or that they and others are all worthwhile, fallible human beings. Some people say that their insight is that they will never blow things out of proportion ever again, or never expect too much of themselves or others again. Everyone has a different summation, a different insight.

Whatever your insight, which technique helped you arrive there? Was it disputing or persuasion? Was it the rational-irrational dialogue, or swearing your beliefs, or a combination of two or more techniques? Which technique do you most identify with, which one is yours?

Again, different people give different answers, for some it's the rationality that disputing gives, for others it's looking at what their beliefs get, others still prefer talking to themselves in a rational-irrational way, and some will forever get a kick out of swearing their beliefs or singing 'Let it Go'.

Whatever answer it is that you give, remember that, in times of trouble, this will be your go-to technique.

Relapse Prevention

Now. What's the difference between a blip and a relapse? And, how do you prevent one from becoming the other?

A blip is an off day. We all have them. A relapse is a return to form. It's you discovering you're back where you were before you ever used REBT.

Blips are inevitable. We all have off days; no one is perfect and everyone is a worthwhile, fallible human being. Don't fear the blip; accept the blip. When a blip occurs, you can either use the tools you have learnt to analyse it, to look at what you told yourself that had you thinking and feeling that way and what you would tell yourself if that situation were to occur again. Or, you can just shrug it off, put it down to an off day, pay it no mind and go to bed on the implicit understanding that tomorrow is another, more rational, day.

At the end of therapy, essentially, there are two types of people who leave the clinic room. Type number one leaves believing, 'Well, I'm in a really good place now. I hope I don't slip up, but I can; I won't like it if I do, but it's not the end of the world; I might find it a challenge if I do, but I know I can cope with that; I am not a failure, even if I slip up, I am a worthwhile, fallible human being.'

These people leave the clinic feeling happy, optimistic and empowered. They understand and accept that blips will occur and that they are part of the process. More importantly, they know what to do if one occurs.

The other type of person leaves the clinic believing, 'Well, I'm in a really good place now, I must not slip up; that would be awful and unbearable and would mean that I have failed.'

These people leave the clinic under pressure; they feel haunted by the potential of a blip. More importantly, if a blip actually occurs, they are more at risk of this developing into a relapse, into a return to form.

So, the main question here is this: having read this book, which sort of person are you going to be?[1]

---

[1] Be the healthy one, be the rational one, don't be the one that says, 'Guess what?'

If you resolve to be the relaxed about the blips sort of person, you're more likely to take things in your stride. It doesn't mean that a relapse will never happen, but it does make one far less likely.

However, if you think you are experiencing a relapse, you are not powerless in the face of it, and there are things you can do. Hopefully, as a result of this book, you have built up a fine body of *Stuff You Did* (i.e. homework). A collection of your thoughts, feelings and beliefs and how you have wrestled with them. Read everything again, from the beginning, adding to it if you need to. If that doesn't work, then go through this book again, from the beginning, as you may have developed a new problem with a new set of unhealthy beliefs.

And, if things get really bad (but not awful, never awful), you can always seek out the services of a professional.

When it comes to people who have seen me before coming back, those who have experienced a relapse (as opposed to those who are simply seeking a 'refresher' session, or who want to work on another problem with a guide), I have one simple question that I ask: 'When did you stop using REBT?'

'How do you know I did?' they often reply.

'Because you are here,' I say. And, nine times out of ten, the answer is the same. They stopped using REBT the moment they left my clinic on the very last session. Mentally, often unconsciously, but rarely on purpose, they just assumed that the job was done and that no more work was needed.

But, the job is never done and REBT is a life-long process. But, as I said, there is no need to be afraid as this process is nowhere near as difficult as it seems.

To prove that point, I want to talk about gardens.[2]

Let's say that you buy a new house. It's a project, a 'fixer upper' and, as you're on a budget, it's you that's going to be doing both the fixing and the upping.

Currently, it has what could technically be called a garden. It's a jungle, though – a mess, overgrown with weeds, full of who-knows-what and a real eyesore. But, you've seen the plans, it's a nice size and, in your mind's eye, you can see how good it could be.

But, to get the jungle looking like that garden in your mind, there's a lot of work that needs to be done; maybe you need to sketch out a plan, maybe not. But, you definitely need to go out there and get your hands dirty. There's weeding to be done, pruning and such-like. You'll probably need to hire a skip to get rid of all the stuff you find lurking in the jungle.

Then, you're off to a garden shop, to buy shrubs and seeds and young plants, which you then plant according to your plan (mental or actual). However, you don't just leave it there, as there's caretaking to be done. You need to protect the seeds and seedlings and so on; you need to water them regularly and keep the cats, caterpillars, slugs, snails and birds off everything.

If you've done your job well, you get up one morning and there you have it, your garden, looking beautiful and just as you imagined it all those weeks ago.

---

[2] The garden as an analogy for change sprouts up in a variety of therapies and for a variety of reasons. This one is a riff of the one taught to me on various courses, including my MSc at Goldsmiths, where the guy that invented it, Windy Dryden, espoused it. All I've done is add garden pests and cat poo.

But, here's the important bit. Now that your garden is looking lovely, do you just leave it alone? Of course you don't. If you do, the weeds will quickly come back, the lawn will become a forest and, all-to-soon, you're back to a jungle again.

So, you need to maintain your garden: a little weeding here, a little pruning there, watering it on a regular basis and scaring the cats off every time you see them about to take a dump on your favourite flower bed.

The question here is this: is any of that maintenance work anywhere near as difficult as clearing it all out and laying it all down in the first place was?

The answer is no; of course not.

I'm hoping the metaphor is clear. Psychologically speaking, we've cleared the garden, planted the seeds, nurtured everything, watched it grow and now your garden is looking lovely. You just need to maintain your gains; you need to come up with little things you can do on a regular basis to prevent the weeds from coming back.[3]

Reading through this book on an occasional basis (or any book on REBT for that matter) would be a good way of maintaining your gains. As would reading through any notes you made and the 'Stuff to Do' you undertook as a result of reading this book.

Some people like to keep an REBT diary or journal. Something they write in on a regular basis. They write down their challenges, especially the ones they don't think they dealt with as well as they would have liked to. They write down what happened, what they told themselves that made them

---

[3] And don't let anyone or anything piddle on anything.

irrational and what they would tell themselves in order to remain rational if that situation were to occur again. They even dig a little deeper into this by adding disputing arguments, or persuasive arguments, to the scenarios and the thoughts that they are sketching out.

More than a fair few people I've seen over the years keep a never-ending rational-irrational dialogue to which they add new challenges and new objections to be worked on and rationalised out.

Another way to maintain your gains is to always keep your language on point. Always use a preference instead of a demand, never use words such as awful, nightmare or ruined, never say something is unbearable or intolerable, and never judge yourself or anyone else as totally useless, rubbish or as a failure. Always use the healthy beliefs in thought and word and deed.

Don't just use them for yourself, or even on yourself. Pass on what you have learnt; drip-feed it to others. We are surrounded by irrationality: at home, at work, even when out socialising with friends. You may even enjoy an elevated social status if you do.

One lady I worked with had very unhealthy beliefs about her life; mainly her lack of academic qualifications and her lacklustre work achievements, but also her then current and long-standing lack of a man. As she put it herself, she was always three or four drinks away from a bit of a meltdown. Which meant that on any given Friday or Saturday night, she could usually be found sobbing on at least one friend's shoulder by the end of it.

All that changed when she began living life according to her healthy beliefs. Her mood improved, she enjoyed her job more than she ever did and she still went out with her friends on a Friday and Saturday night but, instead of wanting a shoulder to cry on, she became *the* shoulder to cry on whenever one of her other friends was distressed. And the advice she gave was now wickedly on point and, more importantly, very rational and all the better for it.

Most people give the same generic, well-intentioned advice, little platitudes that mean well but don't mean much; sayings along the lines of: 'There, there, Julie. You're better than that/them/him/her; there's plenty more fish in the sea; all this will look different tomorrow; just ignore it and it will go away; that's his/her/their loss; they're just jealous, that's all,' and so on, and so on, and so on.

But, now this particular client was dishing out expert REBT advice. Whenever any one of her friends bemoaned the awfulness of their lives, or the intolerable nature of their situation, or expressed demands, or put themselves down, she would pick it apart using the tools and techniques of REBT. Not in a heavy-handed fashion, but conversationally, a dispute there, a persuasion there, a reflection on the healthy alternative to what they said. And she did this, not only with her friends, but also with her family and at work too. And boy, did it make a difference.

'It's been great,' she said, in a follow-up session. 'I'm like a font of knowledge, the wise woman, the sensible one instead of the dramatic one. Everyone turns to me for advice now. And, I absolutely love it.'

More importantly, by passing on what she had learnt on such a regular basis, she was not only helping her friends, family and work colleagues, she was also keeping everything she had learnt about REBT fresh in her mind.

This is what we mean by 'change is a life-long process'. The only way to stay rational about things is to continually think rationally about things while accepting the odd blip here and there.

When you do become a right rational guru and all-round font of REBT knowledge, when you attempt to pass on what you have learnt, it will produce unexpected results, but not always in the way you think. Don't expect it to work on every-body and, more importantly, don't get frustrated with those on whom it does not.

It's an easy mistake to make, you will have learnt to think rationally in the face of adversity, to analyse your thoughts and test them for their validity, their sense and the use. But, not everyone knows what you know. You may attempt to teach them, you may attempt to drip-feed REBT to them and they won't be having any of it. Sometimes, to you, they will sound like squabbling children, and they have every right to be. You may find that difficult to deal with but, like everything else, you can most certainly stand it.

One lady, who I was working with while writing this and who would kill me if she didn't get a mention one way or the other, certainly went through this process. She came to see me with a multitude of problems; anxiety about uncer-tainty, needing to know the outcome of everything; health anxiety, worrying about not being there as her daughter grows up, or something happening to her daughter; not trusting anyone to do anything, as only her way was the right way; problems with her weight, and an unhealthy relationship with food; all linked by a massive dose of the put-downs, evidenced by the belief that she was utterly worthless, useless, ugly and no good. We worked patiently, week by week, step by step and problem by problem until everything changed. She accepted herself, loved herself even, and most definitely loved her life with her husband and her daughter. She stopped hating, started appreciating, and actually experienced moments of pure joy.

It was then that she noticed that people around her were quite demanding (like she used to be); prone to the dramas (as she once was); quite intolerant of pretty much anything (again with the parallels) and, often, if not damning themselves, then definitely very judgemental of others (too close to home for comfort).

She found this difficult for two reasons. Firstly, it reminded her of how she used to be (and she very nearly couldn't stand that); and, secondly, she found their negativity exhausting (and very nearly couldn't stand that either).

So, she tried sharing what she had learnt with the people around her, but that didn't go down too well. Then, she tried drip-feeding it to the same people, but her comments were either ignored at best, or aggressively rebuffed at worst. So, in the end, she simply accepted that as difficult as it was to tolerate these idiosyncrasies, she could deal with them and that it was in her best interests to do so. Plus, she loved these people very much. And, they were all worthwhile, fallible human beings who, more importantly, were on their own journeys and not on hers. She was not responsible for them; she was only responsible for herself. And that was okay. She was a work in progress.

And you are too. Day by day, every day, until thinking in terms of REBT becomes your natural way of thinking. However, even when it does become your natural way of thinking, you will still experience the occasional off day because everyone does, because everyone is a worthwhile, fallible human being. Even the best of therapists occasionally flip out.[4]

As you work on your beliefs, as you move from the rational to the irrational, you will have good days and bad days, you will do better on some days than on others. And, like most things in life, we have an idiom to cover this: 'two steps forwards and one step back'.

Because, life is like that; learning a new language, or a new skill, is like that. Getting to grips with anything is like that; self-improvement is like that. Change is not a linear process. It's a case of two steps forwards and one step back. And that's okay. Don't deny it, accept it – and embrace it even.

Appreciate the successes by all means, but, more importantly, learn from your mistakes. Remember, you are like a scientist or a sportsperson now and, as with all the sciences and all the sports, there are no failures, only opportunities to learn.

Remember the Emerson quote from earlier, that all life is an experiment? Well, now you can experiment with your life.

You are free to experiment with your thoughts and your beliefs using the concepts, tools and techniques of Rational Emotive Behaviour Therapy, the first form of Cognitive Behaviour Therapy, and a therapy that most people have never heard of (including many people who have actually had it as their form of psychotherapy).

I hope it works as well for you as it has for me, and for the many, many people I have seen over the years.

---

[4] This one does.

Frequently Asked Questions

He who asks a question is a fool for five minutes, he who does not ask a question remains a fool forever.

Chinese Proverb

I've included this quote for one very important reason. And the reason is that I do not like this quote. Because there are no fools, there are only worthwhile, fallible human beings. You might ask a clever question, and you might not; you might ask a foolish question, and you might not. But, you are not a fool for asking a foolish question (not even for five minutes). And yet, over the years, I've lost count of the amount of times that proverb has been trolled out at workshops and speaking events. Mainly to put people at their ease when it comes to the Q&A section of their talk. If you have a question, then ask it. If you didn't understand something, seek clarification.

This is very important when talking to an REBT therapist, or any therapist for that matter. Never be afraid to ask a question, never let your therapist assume you've understood something when you haven't, and never simply nod and say 'yes' when asked if you have understood something and you haven't. All questions are important questions and there are no fools, only foolish things. And not asking a question when you need to know the answer is a very foolish thing indeed. The following are some fairly common questions that people ask of REBT.

Can I Really Solve All My Problems in Just Six Sessions?

No, you can get control over one problem, as long as it is a specific problem, in just six sessions. I'm not comfortable with words such as 'cure' or 'solve' and would advise you to shy away from therapists that say they can cure you, or solve your problems. Better to seek out a therapist that says they can help you gain control. This book can help you gain control over a specific problem. So, if you are angry with your partner over a specific aspect of your relationship, if you are anxious about giving presentations at work, if you are jealous around your new partner because your previous partner wasn't trustworthy, if you are still depressed because of that job you lost, then I am confident that you can resolve that problem in six sessions as long as you apply yourself diligently to the homework required at each stage.

However, if you have more than one problem, the model still stands. It's just that, once you've arrived at the E in the ABCDE model of psychological health (which stands for Effective rational outlook), it just means that you work on another problem according to the same model, with the same tools (while still monitoring where you are with the previous problem).[1]

But, What If I Can't Fix My Problems In Just Six Sessions; What If I Am Struggling With This Book?

This is a self-help therapy book and, I hope, an efficacious one, but it's no substitute for an experienced therapist, especially if you're struggling with some complicated stuff. However, don't give up just yet. As mentioned previously, six sessions is sufficient if your problem is specific and at the mild to moderate end of the spectrum. It also helps to have a clear goal in mind. That said, each session needs to go according to plan for the 'six sessions' to hold. And, for many people, things do indeed go according to plan. But, things do not go according to plan for everyone and, even when they do, they don't do it all the time.

If you feel this is happening to you, for whatever reason, it doesn't mean that this book has failed you or that you have failed at it (both are worthwhile and fallible). Some people take to REBT like the proverbial duck to water. For others, it's a completely new and complicated way of thinking and so, in their experience, it's like chucking a spanner into the well-oiled engine of their mind and watching everything go 'clunk!' All this means is that you might have to repeat one or two of the chapters once or twice. If you don't think you've understood

---

[1] This applies, not only to multiple problems, but also to multiple emotions in the face of the same problem.

disputing or persuasion, then go back to those chapters. If you go to put your learning into practice but falter, if you still get anxious or angry, then go back to the rational-irrational dialogue, as you may still have a few objections to iron out before you're ready. Don't expect to be perfect first time, plan for a strong negative emotion, even when it's healthy, and accept that you need to repeat your behavioural tasks as often as possible for the intensity of the emotion to abate. Don't forget, there are no failures, only opportunities to learn. Think of your behavioural tasks as experiments. You may get the results you want first time, and you may not. If you don't, you simply analyse the results, tweak things as necessary and repeat until you get the desired outcome. Six weeks could become eight or 10 that way, but you'll still be doing some really good work.

Surely, There Are More Than Just Four Thoughts, Though?

Yes, there are. Experts estimate that the mind is thinking somewhere between 60,000 and 80,000 thoughts a day, which is an average of 2,500 to 3,300 thoughts per hour. And most of them are superfluous, or are thoughts we barely notice. According to REBT, the four thoughts that fuck you up are four specific beliefs, held in the face of a specific problem. All other dysfunctional thoughts, feelings, behaviours and symptoms about that problem are but consequences of those four beliefs. When you change those four beliefs to their rational counterparts, all your other thoughts about that problem will, naturally, become more rational too.

Isn't Rational Emotive Behaviour Therapy All A Bit Too Repetitive?

Yes, definitely, and importantly, so. We learn through repetition. Just think about how you learnt your times tables at school, or how you revised for any test or exam. Repetition is key to our learning. With REBT you repeat exercises such as disputing, persuasive arguments and rational-irrational dialogues over and over again to effect a shift from one belief system to the other. When you can feel that shift take place, you then need to act in accordance with that healthy belief, not once or twice, not a few times, but repeatedly, over and over again, until that shift becomes permanent. Don't shy away from the repetition, embrace it.

Isn't REBT Too Simplistic?

It could be seen that way but REBT therapists prefer the term 'elegant'. Back in the day, when it was just a fledgling therapy, REBT had more than four thoughts to fuck you up, more like twenty or so but, over the years the therapy has been refined and refined. It's not saying that people aren't complicated, because they are; and it's not saying that problems are simple to solve, because they're not. In fact, problems can become so complicated that they create problems of their own and then we disturb ourselves about those problems in a myriad of new and unhealthy ways.

The first time I ever went to therapy, I sat down in front of the therapist, outlined the issue that had brought me there but, then, started to discuss my entire (quite colourful) personal history, just to help paint a picture. After a while, I stopped, mainly because of the horrified look on her face.

'You're a little bit out of your depth, aren't you?' I asked. She nodded in nervous acquiescence.

'I'm going to have to consult my supervisor,' she said.

'I'd prefer it if I saw your supervisor for the next session then please.'

'Oh you will definitely be seeing someone else,' she said with relief.

The next week, my new therapist explained my problems using (what I later learnt) was the ABCDE model of psychological health. It was my first ever introduction to it, in fact.

It's an excellent model, as it helps to take complicated things and break them down into more workable scenarios.

You use that model to work on a single, specific problem. Problem by problem, one by one. We don't tackle everything *en masse* as that would just complicate things. With REBT, you can take the most interlocked Gordian knot of problems and begin to tease them out, one by one, strand by strand.

With the ABCDE model, you know where you are and what you are doing, every step of the way.

I Have More Than One Problem; I Probably Have Dozens Of Problems. Does This Mean I Will Be Using This Book, Or Be in Therapy, Forever?

I hope not. All forms of CBT are considered to be brief therapies, which means you're with a therapist for weeks to months, as opposed to months to years. With REBT, the idea is that, at some point, just by working on a few problems, you make a profound philosophical shift in the way you look at life and all of your problems. Not only that, but things are more connected than they seem. Your problems are like trees. No, really, I'm serious.

Do you know any tree surgeons? If not, do you know what a tree surgeon does? Basically, a tree surgeon fixes trees. They help preserve old and damaged trees. Now, let's say you're walking through a forest and you spy a large clump of sickly looking trees. You might think that the tree surgeon has their work cut out for them. But, the tree surgeon knows something you may not. They only have to work on one tree, maybe the sickliest one, and as they work on it, it will have a healing effect on many of the trees immediately surrounding it. So, by working on one, they are in fact working on many, because things are more connected than they seem. Three or four trees later, and the whole clump is healed. Your problems are a lot like those trees. You could have a problem list a hundred problems long. But, as you work on one, you will be pleasantly surprised at how many other problems will be resolved as a result. So, by all means, come up with as big a list as you think you need, but don't be put off by it.[2]

---

[2] I have asked two actual tree surgeons if this analogy is correct, just to be sure. One said, 'Yes, definitely,' and the other said 'Yes, sort of.' So phew, and sort of phew, then.

Will I Be Giving Up The Things That Are Important To Me?

People often ask this one. Especially people who like to be in control of things, or who are perfectionists. REBT does not seek to take someone who cares about something and then turn him or her into someone who doesn't care about something. When we are disturbed, the problem isn't that we care, it's that we care far too much, more than is healthy or rational. REBT just helps you to dial it back down. You still care, and maybe care a lot, but not so much that you disturb yourself. Take perfectionism, for instance. There are people who just don't care about things being 'just so', who just aren't bothered by being slap-dash or half-assed about work projects and such-like. If you were to quiz them on it, you would probably find that their belief system is either 'I don't care about perfection' or 'I neither care nor don't care about perfection'. Someone who has the demand 'everything I do must be perfect' will go out of his, her or their way to ensure that things are prefect. They won't just push themselves, they will push themselves too far. They will push themselves over the edge. Someone who believes 'I prefer everything I do to be perfect, but I know it doesn't have to be' still cares about perfection because that is their preference. As they care, they will still push themselves, because they are motivated by that preference, but they will not be pushing themselves over the edge.[3]

---

[3] If it helps, you can say, 'I really, really strongly prefer everything I do to be perfect, but I also know it doesn't have to be (because it can't, not always).'

REBT Seems Very Verbal And Very Wordy. I Am Neither, So Does This Mean That REBT Is Not For Me?

Well, hopefully, you won't have found reading this book or undertaking the assignments it has set too taxing but, if you have, there are other approaches. While it's true that all forms of CBT are known as 'talking therapies', it's also true that you can tailor the homework to an approach that suits you best. Not everything has to be wordy and not everything has to be written. Over the years, I've had plenty of people use the voice memo function on their smart phones to dispute their beliefs and develop persuasive arguments verbally, in their language, not mine; in a way that makes sense to them, not me. I've had plenty of people record the actual session in the same way and simply play it back to themselves. Other people have taken homework assignments similar to those set in this book and used their tablets and laptops to turn them into graphs, charts, storyboards, mood boards, visual diaries and more. I've also had more than a fair few people turn what they learnt in session and what was set for them as homework into mind maps, as that's what worked best for them. One memorable client bought a stack of file cards and a file box and wrote one pertinent point on each file card and would go through the stack on a regular basis. You don't have to do the assignments set in this book as I have described them, feel free to take what you have learnt and put them into a form that both makes sense to you and helps you work on your beliefs.[4]

---

[4] An Emoji-based piece of homework is out there, somewhere, I'm sure.

Will I Become An Emotionless Robot If I Use This Therapy?

This. Does not. Compute. Yes, REBT contains the word 'rational' in its name, and yes, we employ logic in helping you rationalise your beliefs, but we don't mean logic like a robot or like a Vulcan (for you *Star Trek* fans out there). In REBT every single unhealthy negative emotion has a healthy negative counterpart. Don't forget, unhealthy simply means unhelpful to you and/or others, while healthy means helpful to you and/or others. When you hold unhealthy beliefs you think and feel and act in ways that don't actually help you but, when you hold healthy beliefs, you think and feel and act in ways that are helpful to you. Acting and reacting without emotion is neither healthy nor helpful. Sometimes you will have things to be concerned about, or sad about, or frustrated about. More importantly, those emotions will exist on a scale (say from a little bit concerned to very concerned indeed). The more concerning a thing is, the more concerned you will be but, as long as your beliefs are healthy, then no matter how intensely you feel the emotion, it will be healthy so your thoughts and behaviours will be equally healthy (i.e. helpful to you). Us Brits used to be famous for something called 'The Stiff Upper Lip'. Most people thought it meant that we were very good at repressing our emotions to the point where we became spectacularly insane, but actually, it's better than that. A person with a stiff upper lip displays fortitude and stoicism in the face of adversity or exercises great self-restraint in the expression of emotion (or, at least according to Wikipedia, it does). And that is the essence of REBT. It's a therapy that helps you develop that fortitude and stoicism and, while doing so, it most definitely wants you to express your emotions, but it wants you to express them appropriately.

Surely Events Do Cause Emotions Though, Especially When It's Something Really Traumatic?

When something really traumatic happens, you are allowed to be traumatised and, at that point CBT may not be the best tool in the therapy tool box. Counselling, which just offers you a safe space in which to speak, might be a bitter fit for you at this point. That said, there is such a thing as trauma-focussed CBT and I have certainly worked a lot with people who are traumatised.

If you've made it through this book, I am hoping that you understand that when something happens, it will influence the way you think and feel and act, but only influence. And that, more directly, it's your beliefs about the event that truly determine how you think and feel and act. Now, the more traumatic an event is, the more of an influence over your emotions and behaviours it will be.

Let's say that you are involved in an accident, or are a survivor of domestic abuse or sexual assault. These are very clearly Activating events at A in the ABCDE model of psychological health. Now, in the aftermath of the event, in the immediacy of it, you are allowed to be all kinds of disturbed, you are allowed to be all 'should' and 'shouldn't'. What you need is time to recover, to process and to heal; to move on. With time, your demands will naturally become preferences. REBT is the tool to use if that doesn't happen. If you're still stuck with your demands months or even years after the traumatic incident, then you need to look at your beliefs. But, the principle of emotional responsibility: that it's not the events in life that disturb you, but what you tell yourself about those events that disturbs you, still stands.

If I Accept My Healthy Beliefs About Myself and Other People, Am I Letting Myself (Or Those Others) Off The Hook When We Do Bad Things?

I really hope not. I am hoping that when it comes to yourself, you are holding a belief along the lines of 'I wish I hadn't done that bad thing, but there is no reason why I mustn't have, I'm not a bad person, even though I did a bad thing, I am a worthwhile, fallible human being'. You will still experience an emotion with that belief, and it won't be a happy one; it will be a healthy negative emotion, with appropriate behaviours attached. More importantly, you are clearly stating that there was a bad thing, and that you wish you hadn't done it; but that doing bad doesn't make you completely bad. This doesn't let you off the hook at all. With it, you will prefer to do good because you wish you hadn't done bad, you might have to atone with what you did, and live with what you did, but you can move on from it in a healthy and constructive way. It's the same with other people.

You are not accepting them as worthwhile, fallible human beings to let them off the hook; you are doing it to get yourself off a hook (anger is a hook, depression is a hook and so on).

However, forgiving someone who has wronged you, accepting them as a worthwhile and fallible human being, doesn't mean you have to accept them back into your life. If someone has become toxic for you, you have every right to tell them to sling their hook, to bugger right off out of your life, but you say so while accepting them and wishing them well with the rest of their life (as long as that life is conducted far, far away from you).

Is REBT Better Than CBT Or Vice Versa?

The short answer is no. All forms of CBT attempt to do the same thing, albeit from slightly different angles, perspectives and philosophies. Many people have come to me over the years and said something along the lines of, 'I wish I'd had this form of CBT years ago,' or, 'I've had both forms of CBT and I much prefer this one.' But, I am sure that many people have come to CBT saying the exact same things about REBT.

The Aaron T. Beck CBT model is more prevalent than the Albert Ellis REBT model, and that is something I really hope this book addresses. Why that is so is kind of complicated. Many therapists and academics say it's because Beck was quicker to realise the importance of backing his therapy up with scientific research (i.e. evidence). But, I have other ideas.

For me, it's like the battle between HD-DVD and Blu-Ray. Both technologies hit the market at the same time. Both were equal in terms of sound and vision quality. But, Blu-Ray won the fight through slicker marketing and a cooler name. It captured the public consciousness quicker and stayed there.

Going back a little further along the home entertainment time-line, we had the battle between VHS video and Betamax (now, I am showing my age). Technically, Betamax was the superior product (and here, I cast no CBT aspersions); it had better technology and superior sound and vision quality, but VHS won the day, possibly due to slicker marketing but, also because it simply caught the public consciousness first. Plus, it was a bit cheaper.

I would like REBT to be very much back in the public consciousness, because this isn't home entertainment, it's psychotherapy and, if there is a form of it that suits you better, you should know about it and should be able to ask for it and access it.

As a famous former Victoria's Secret Angel once said, 'I feel like knowledge is power. If you know how to take care of yourself you can be a better version of yourself.'[5]

---

[5] Australian model, Miranda May Kerr.

In Conclusion

Nothing ever goes away until it has taught us what we need to know.

Pema Chödrön

So, there you have it. A book about Rational Emotive Behaviour Therapy: a system of psychotherapy that's widely accepted as the first form of Cognitive Behaviour Therapy, and a very successful and long-standing form of it at that. Sadly, it is also one that not enough people outside the field of psychotherapy have heard of.

Books about REBT have been written before. Many of them, in fact, but not as many people who could be aware of them are aware of them.

More people are aware of, say, *Mind Over Mood* by Christine Padesky, than are aware of, say, *Reason to Change* by Windy Dryden. And yet, to my mind, *Reason to Change* is the much better offering, especially if you are mechanically minded. If you are, then *Reason to Change* is like a Haynes Manual for the brain.[1]

---

[1] Or a 'partworks' magazine collection only, you're not building a model Batmobile or Millennium Falcon, you're building a new you.

REBT is not a therapy of my own devising; the ABCDE model of psychological health is not my model. All I have done here is taken the methods, therapy and philosophy of Albert Ellis, as they were taught to me, and taken them out for a spin of my own. I hope you enjoyed the ride. I hope I've encouraged you to find out more.

There is nothing new under the sun. The latest buzzwords in CBT are acceptance and commitment therapy (ACT) and compassion focussed therapy (CFT); both of which are very fine modalities. Both have a slightly different focus than both REBT and CBT and have added mindfulness to the offering.

Mindfulness is based on *ancient* Buddhist practice, and the architects of REBT and CBT both acknowledge the role that *ancient* Stoic philosophy played in the therapies they built. Emphasis is on the *ancient* here, because there is nothing new under the sun. Everything that is considered 'new' is also considered to be somehow 'superior' to what has gone before. But, CBT is not better than REBT and ACT and CFT are not better than either CBT or REBT and, while mindfulness and mindfulness-based therapies are both brilliant, neither are they the be-all-and-end-all of therapeutic practices.[2]

Nothing is. Including REBT. A lot of it comes down to who you are, how you process information and how ready for change you are at the time. It also depends on how much effort you're willing to put in. Mindfulness works best when you practice it every day. The same can be said for Rational Emotive Behaviour Therapy.

---

[2] For fans of the 'double whammy', you can get mindfulness based cognitive therapy (MBCT) and mindfulness based REBT (MBREBT).

Everyone is looking for a quick fix and everyone is looking for the therapy that will fix them quickly. Psychologists and researchers alike are looking for the therapeutic equivalent of the Unified Theory of Everything. Or, a magic wand, where one wave or one session fixes all.[3]

Maybe, one day, they will even find it. However, it's human nature that, in the rush for the new, we not only forget the old, but also the recent. In looking for The Next Big Thing, we drop what Was Still A Good Thing.[4]

I would hate to see REBT go the way of the dodo, or become so sublimated into other therapies that it dilutes into nothing, or becomes something it wasn't. It probably will, even Albert Ellis, when asked what he thought would happen to REBT, predicted that it would probably be subsumed into other therapies, or watered-down even, to the point where it disappeared. But, let's not give up just yet.

Other people haven't. Several Albert Ellis titles were re-released only last year, so perhaps there is a resurgent interest in the subject. I hope so. It never quite had its heyday. And by heyday, I mean it never seeped into the public consciousness

---

[3] Single Session Therapy (SST) is a thing; and it's even a thing offered by Professor Windy Dryden who was one of the people who taught me REBT, but SST is not a magic wand and will still require much effort on your part.

[4] We've all been there. We've all dumped someone for someone else, someone new and shiny and more alluring, and then realized that the previous someone was way better for us than the current someone. As it is with relationships, so too is it with therapy and therapists.

enough that they knew it was an option. But, it is very much an option and a most marvellous option at that.

Over the years, so many people have come into my practice and group therapy sessions and, after just a few sessions or so, or by the end of therapy, have said, 'I wish I'd known about this therapy sooner.'

Despite REBT having been around since the mid-1950s, despite there being many books on the subject, so many have told me, 'I wish I'd known about this therapy years ago. My life would have been so different if I had.'

If you have read this book, then you are aware of REBT and you can pass that knowledge on to your friends. You or they could enquire about it when looking for the best-fit therapy for yourselves; you could not only ask if your potential therapist had CBT skills, but also REBT skills; you could ask if your healthcare provider provided REBT, or if REBT is available via your local NHS trust. You could even feel empowered enough to learn this style of therapy for yourselves. Nothing reassures quite like knowledge and choice. Not everyone who chooses to learn CBT even knows about REBT, or knows that it is a form of CBT.

If you want to pursue REBT as your therapy of choice, not every REBT therapist advertises themselves as one, but you can access the Association of Rational Emotive Behaviour Therapists (AREBT) or the British Association for Behavioural & Cognitive Psychotherapies (BABCP) to find a practising REBT therapist near you.

And, if you would like to study the subject yourself, either as a form of self-help or to learn how to become an REBT therapist in your own right, I can heartily recommend the

College of Cognitive Behavioural Therapies (CCBT) which runs courses in both London and Bath (in the Southwest of England) and there's the Centre for Rational Emotive Behaviour Therapy at the University of Birmingham. It's the UK affiliate of the Albert Ellis Institute in New York which, in turn, is the international home of all things REBT. Also, the Centre for Stress Management in London runs excellent and approved courses.

And talking of stress, I just cannot stress enough how effective REBT is, not only at managing specific problems, but also at looking at life in a whole new way.

But, when it comes to those pesky specific problems, people always ask, 'How many sessions will this take?' And, when I say, 'Six sessions for you,' they nearly always exclaim, 'What? Really? Six sessions?'

And the answer is yes.

If you have one specific problem, the answer is yes; if you are motivated and committed to the process, the answer is yes and, if you do your homework to the best of your ability, the answer is yes.

In fact, when I practised in London, where people are very focussed on quick fixes, most of the people I saw were in and out in just six sessions. The hardest part of being a self-employed REBT therapist in London was finding new clients to replace the rapidly departing old ones.

We would whizz, not only through the ABCDE model of psychological health, but all the exercises in this book (and others like them) rapidly, and to very good effect.

I was always keen to point out that the therapy that had just helped them so rapidly and effectively was called REBT.

For me, those letters stand as much for the process of therapy as they do for the type of therapy – each letter means something in the same way that each letter of the ABCDE model stands for something.

People come to therapy because they are irrational. They are thinking and feeling and acting in ways that they don't like, but can't seem to change. The technical term for this is 'neurosis', which means they are suffering from a relatively mild mental illness that is not caused by any organic disease. These people are also known as 'the worried well', although the term itself can seriously belie the severity of the symptoms the sufferer experiences. But, it also means, by definition, that the sufferer generally hasn't lost touch with reality. This is as opposed to psychosis, which means someone has a mental disorder so severe that thoughts and emotions are so impaired that those people have indeed lost touch with reality.

So, people arrive irrational, they arrive as the worried well. As an REBT therapist, we first need to get them Rational. We teach them to analyse and challenge the validity of their thoughts. We then get them to use more Emotive techniques to undermine their unhealthy beliefs and build a conviction in their healthy beliefs. When this conviction is high enough, they need to Behave according to their healthy beliefs as much as possible and for the rest of their lives. It is only by repeatedly behaving according to our healthy beliefs that we can achieve our therapeutic goals.

Not all therapists set goals, as not all therapies are goal-directed. But, bearing in mind that people are, by nature, goal-directed, it makes such good sense to have a therapy that offers that.[5]

I hope this book has helped you to achieve yours.

My goal all those years ago was to not shout, swear or make animal noises at the people who bumped into me in crowded places. That mission was accomplished, more or less. Because, these days, and to paraphrase a well-used dating app trope, I don't growl.

Unless you want me to, that is.

---

[5] People tend to feel a little listless and lacklustre if they don't have goals.

Acknowledgements

I am massively indebted to all the people who taught me Rational Emotive Behaviour Therapy. Mainly because I've loved it so much. Indirectly there was Albert Ellis, the founding father of the subject while, directly, there was Avy Joseph, co-founder of the College of Cognitive Behavioural Therapies (who first introduced me to the subject when running his cognitive behavioural hypnotherapy diploma course) and, later Professor Windy Dryden (who also taught Avy) and Rhena Branch who both taught me on the MSc at Goldsmith's College, University of London. Three Yodas to my Luke Skywalker: All together they taught me the structure, processes and intricacies of REBT both thoroughly and well. The idiosyncrasies and slight deviations from the norm contained within this book, however, are all of my own. Sorry about that, people!

My thanks go also to my agent Robert Gwyn Palmer (for some top agenting), and to Susanna Abbott (for saying 'yes'), and to Emma Owen, Kate Latham and all at Penguin Random House who helped bring this book to fruition.

Resources

College of Cognitive Behavioural Therapies (CCBT)

www.cbttherapies.org.uk

Association of Rational Emotive Behavioural Therapy (AREBT)

www.arebt.eu

British Association for Behavioural & Cognitive Psychotherapies (BABCP)

www.babcp.com

Centre for Stress Management (CSM)

www.managingstress.com

Centre for Rational Emotive Behaviour Therapy – University of Birmingham

www.birmingham.ac.uk

Albert Ellis Institute

www.albertellis.org

Further Reading

Dryden, Windy, *Reason to Change: A Rational Emotive Behaviour Therapy Workbook*, (2001, Routledge)

Dryden, Windy, *Ten Steps to Positive Living*: New Edition, (2014, Sheldon Press)

Ellis, Albert, *How to Make Yourself Happy and Remarkably Less Disturbable*, (New edition 1999, Impact)

Ellis, Albert, *How to Stubbornly Refuse to Make Yourself Miserable: About Anything – Yes, Anything!* (New edition 2019, Robinson)

Joseph, Avy & Chapman, Maggie, *Confidence and Success with CBT: Small Steps to Achieve Your Big Goals with Cognitive Behaviour Therapy* (2013, Capstone)

Joseph, Avy & Chapman, Maggie, *Visual CBT: Using Pictures to Help you Apply Cognitive Behaviour Therapy*, (2013, Capstone)

INDEX

INDEX

Grande, Ariana: 'Problem' 282
gravity, law of 17–18, 26
grief counselling 10
Grumpus 1, 1n
guilt 63–4, 100, 161, 163, 171–2, 176, 178
gym 55–6, 60, 115, 116

Harry Potter franchise 269
Hauck, Dr Paul 67, 127
Health and Safety Executive (HSE) 51
healthy thoughts, four *see* four healthy
    thoughts
hierarchy of needs, human 273–4
high frustration tolerance (HFT) *see*
    'I can copes'/high frustration
    tolerance (HFT)
Hitler, Adolf 123–5, 124n, 128
homework 10, 49, 127, 155–6, 214,
    216, 238, 251n, 254, 255, 256,
    265, 268, 270, 275, 279, 280,
    287, 296, 303, 303n, 313
humanistic (or client-centred)
    approach to therapy 261
humour viii, 9, 10, 109n, 119, 224,
    260, 262–3
hurt 70, 72, 163, 172, 173, 174, 176
hypnotherapy 2–3, 69, 252–3

'I can copes'/high frustration tolerance
    (HFT) 108–19, 133, 188, 191,
    199, 210–11, 232; four types of
    'I can't cope' and 118–19; idioms
    that encapsulate 108–9, 109n,
    114; 'I will find this thing tedious,
    or boring, but I know I can be
    bothered'/'while I find this
    information difficult to process, I
    can believe it' 114–15
'I can't copes'/low frustration
    tolerance (LFT) v, 45–61,
    107, 185, 186, 198, 214, 230;
    achievement intolerance and 52,
    118; discomfort intolerance and
    52, 118; disputing and 57–61;
    emotional intolerance and 52,
    118; entitlement intolerance

and 52, 118; flipping your buts
    and 55–6, 115; four types of 52,
    118–19; 'I can't be bothered' and
    'I can't believe it' 53–4, 55, 60–1,
    114–16; 'I can't deal with that
    right now' 45; 'unbelievable' as
    a low frustration tolerance belief
    54–5
ideal demands 18–19
idioms 38, 95, 108–9, 109n, 114, 294
instant gratification 50
intellectual understanding vii, 216
irrational language 271–5

jealousy 8, 9, 20, 159, 163, 169–70,
    171n, 175–6, 291, 296
judgement: by other people 97, 179,
    180, 183, 184, 185, 186, 187,
    188, 189, 201–5, 219–20, 223–8,
    238–46, 261, 266, 293; judging
    others 73, 75, 293; judging
    yourself 65, 68, 69–70, 89, 121,
    130, 227–8, 241, 242, 244, 245,
    246

Keele University 264

laughter 262–3
Lord of the Rings, The 266–8, 269
loser, judging yourself as a 65, 68,
    69–70, 89, 121, 130, 227–8, 241,
    242, 244, 245, 246
low frustration tolerance (LFT) *see*
    'I can't copes'/low frustration
    tolerance (LFT)

Malcolm X 81
Maslow, Abraham: 'A Theory of Human
    Motivation' 273
mindfulness 310, 310n
Murakami, Haruki 114

National Health Service (NHS) 8–9,
    312
National Institute of Clinical Excellence
    (NICE) guidelines 8–9